ELEVENTH EDITION

Self-Therapy
for the
Stutterer

By

Malcolm Fraser, L.H.D.

Life Member
American Speech-Language-Hearing Association

Founder
Stuttering Foundation of America

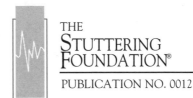

THE
STUTTERING
FOUNDATION®

PUBLICATION NO. 0012

self-therapy for the stutterer

Publication No. 0012

First Edition—1978
Tenth Edition—2002
Revised Tenth Edition—2007
Eleventh Edition—2010
Second Printing—2017

Published by

Stuttering Foundation of America
Post Office Box 11749
Memphis, Tennessee 38111-0749

Library of Congress Control Number: 2010932952
ISBN 978-0-933388-93-2

Printed in the United States of America.

Dedicated to all
who seek relief from the burden
of stuttering.

To the Reader

There are always some stutterers who are unable to get professional help and others who do not seem to be able to profit from it. There are some who prefer to be their own therapists. In this book, Malcolm Fraser, Founder of the Stuttering Foundation of America, has provided some guidance for those who must help themselves. Knowing well from his own experience as a stutterer the difficulties of self-therapy, he outlines a series of objectives and challenges that should serve as a map for the person who is lost in the dismal swamp of stuttering and wants to find a way out.

CHARLES VAN RIPER

Distinguished Professor Emeritus and formerly Head, Department of Speech Pathology and Audiology, Western Michigan University

"The stutterer must conquer his own problems. No one else can do it for him."

—Van Riper

Contents

*Use the Index (page 189) for location of instructive
information concerning all phases of stuttering*

The person who stutters in this book is often referred to as "he" or "him." This is done for editorial reasons but may be considered as fairly representative since it is estimated that 3 to 4 times as many males stutter as females.

The quotations and footnotes in this book have been taken from the writings of speech-language pathologists and medical doctors. All of them have earned degrees as doctors of philosophy or medicine and know what you are up against as most stutter themselves. They understand your problem from observation and experience and represent a most distinguished array of authority and prestige in the field of stuttering. Their names and titles are listed starting on page 186. Those who stutter are marked with a star by their name.

———————

"The importance of motivation cannot be exaggerated, and success or failure of therapy will depend on your commitment to follow through."

———————

———————

In case you are not familiar with the meanings of some of the words used in this book, you will find a glossary beginning on page 171 where definitions are given of terms and expressions used in the treatment of stuttering including many not found in this book. Read them for your general education in speech pathology.

———————

On Self-Therapy

If you are like many of the three million stutterers in this country, adequate clinical treatment will not be available to you. Whatever you do you'll have to be pretty much on your own with what ideas and resources you can use. (Sheehan)

The first thing you must do is to admit to yourself that you need to change, that you really want to do something about the way you presently talk. This is tough but your commitment must be total; not even a small part of you must hold back. Don't dwell longingly on your fluency in the magical belief that some day your speech blocks will disappear. There is no magic potion, no pink pill that will cure stuttering.

Don't sit around waiting for the right time for inspiration to come to you—*you must go to it.* You must see that the old solutions, the things you have done to help yourself over the years simply do not work. Ruts wear deep though, and you will find it difficult to change. Even though the way you presently talk is not particularly pleasant, it is familiar. It is the unknown from which we shrink.

You must be willing to endure temporary discomfort, perhaps even agony, for the long range improvement you desire. No one is promising you a rose garden. Why not take the time and effort now for a lifetime of freedom from your tangled tongue? How can you do this? Break down the global problem of stuttering into its parts and then solve them one at a time. No one said it was easy. Shall we begin?
(Emerick)

A valuable precondition for a successful therapy is the deep inner conviction of the stutterer in the manageability of his disorder, combined with a fighting spirit and a readiness to undergo hardships and deprivations if needed— hopelessness, pessimism and passivity being the deadliest foes to self-improvement. *(Freund)*

"There is no quick and easy way to tackle stuttering, but with the right approach, self-therapy can be effective."

On This Approach to Self-Therapy

This book is written to and for the many adults and teenagers who stutter[1,3]—and is addressed in the second person to describe what you can and should do to control your stuttering. We state confidently that as a stutterer, you do not need to surrender helplessly to your speech difficulty because you can change the way you talk. You can learn to communicate with ease rather than with effort. There is no quick and easy way to tackle stuttering, but with the right approach, self-therapy can be effective.

Experience may have caused you to be skeptical about any plan which claims to offer a solution. You may have tried different treatment ideas and been disappointed and disillusioned in the past. This book promises no quick magical cure and makes no false claims.[2] It describes what you can and should do to build self-confidence and overcome your difficulty.

It offers a logical practical program of therapy based on methods and procedures that have been used successfully in many universities and other speech clinics. This approach to therapy has been shown to get results.[3] If there were an easier or better way of learning how to control stuttering, we would recommend it.

---

[1]Almost one percent of the population of this country manifest some acute form of stuttering speech, which places them under a great economic and social handicap. This can be corrected if given the proper training. (Martin)

[2]There are no quick or magical answers to your stuttering. (Barbara)

[3]*Self Therapy* has been translated into no less than 26 languages including: Lithuanian, Czech, Zulu, Japanese, Chinese, French, Spanish, Portuguese, Italian, Russian, Arabic, Cambodian, Vietnamese, Persian, Icelandic, Slovakian, Finnish, Danish, Swedish, Flemish, Swahili, Solvenian, Greek, and more.

We start with two assumptions. One is that you have no physical defect or impairment of your speech mechanism that will get in the way of your achieving more fluent speech. After all, you can probably talk without stuttering when you are alone or not being heard or observed by others.[1,2] Practically all those who stutter have periods of fluency, and most speak fluently part of the time.

> "You are the only person on earth who can correct your stuttering."
>
> —Starbuck

And we assume that you may not be in a position to avail yourself of the services of a speech pathologist, trained to help you work on your problem in the manner described in this book and that, as a result, you need to be your own therapist. Even with competent guidance, authorities would agree that stuttering therapy is largely a do-it-yourself project anyway.[3,4,5,6]

If you are sincerely interested in working on your speech, you will need to have a strong motivation to overcome your difficulty and a sincere determination to follow through on the suggested procedures and assignments.

---

[1]There is nothing wrong inside your body that will stop you from talking. You have the ability to talk normally. (D. Williams)

[2]Because you stutter doesn't mean you are biologically inferior to the next person. (Sheehan)

[3]No one but myself improved my speech. Others have helped me by providing information, giving emotional support, identifying bias, etc. but the dirty work of therapy is, and always has been, my responsibility. (Boehmler)

[4]Don't ever forget that even if you went to the most knowledgeable expert in the country, the correction of stuttering is a do-it-yourself project. Stuttering is your problem. The expert can tell you what to do and how to do it, but you are the one who has to do it. You are the only person on earth who can correct your stuttering. (Starbuck)

[5]The stutterer must conquer his own problems—no one else can do the job for him. (Van Riper)

[6]Needless to say, each stutterer must from the beginning of therapy accept the responsibility for his problem. This implies self-therapy which is essential. (Stromsta)

The importance of motivation cannot be exaggerated, and success or failure of therapy will depend on your commitment to follow through.[1] It will not be easy, but it can be done.

On the other hand, there is no way to promise success in this or any other program since no sure 'cure' for stuttering has yet been discovered in spite of what you may have read.

However, it is reasonable to believe that if you follow the suggestions and carry out the procedures outlined in this book, you should be able to control your stuttering and speak easily without abnormality. Others have conquered their stuttering and you can too.

But the best way for you to judge the effectiveness of any therapy is to try it out and let the results speak for themselves.[2,3]

The importance of motivation cannot be exaggerated

It should be mentioned that there are many differences among stutterers. Some cases are mild and others severe, and in most cases the frequency and severity of stuttering tends to vary from time to time and from one situation to another.

Sometimes you may be able to speak in a comparatively fluent manner with little or no difficulty; at other times you may have considerable trouble, particularly when the message to be conveyed is important. That tends to make

[1]The importance of motivation cannot be exaggerated. (Hulit)

[2]A major problem in the treatment of stuttering is how to encourage the stutterer to stay in and continue with the course of treatment. (Barbara)

[3]Based on your understanding choose the most appropriate therapy program you can, and work at the program with more consistency, devotion and energy than any other task you've ever tackled. As success is obtained, maintain it with equal vigor. (Boehmler)

it a most frustrating disorder since it can and usually does become worse in certain environments and under certain circumstances.

Most stutterers are apt to have the most difficulty when embarrassed and anticipating trouble.[1] As one person expressed it, "if you can't afford to stutter, you will."

...if you can't afford to stutter, you will.

It may be more noticeable when you are asked to state your name, when talking to people in authority like prospective employers, teachers, in making introductions, when speaking to groups or talking on the telephone, etc. On the other hand, you may have little or no trouble when talking to yourself or talking to a child or a pet animal.[2]

It should also be recognized that stutterers vary widely in their reactions and characteristics and in the conditions under which their stuttering occurs. No two persons stutter in the same manner since every stutterer has developed his own particular pattern of stuttering.[3,4,5] All those who stutter have a wide variety of personality traits, so your reactions may be different from others; and accord-

---

[1]Stuttering is an anticipatory struggle reaction. (Bloodstein)

[2]Some stutterers have difficulty reading aloud; others do not. Some can speak well when in a position of authority; some show their greatest difficulty here. Some can use the telephone without interference; others are completely frustrated by this situation. Speaking with members of the opposite sex causes great difficulty to one stutterer but results in fluency with another. Some speak well at home but not in other environments; with others the situation is completely reversed. (Ansberry)

[3]The old saying that no two stutterers are alike is undoubtedly true. (Luper)

[4]The speech behavior patterns that have usually been associated with or identified as stuttering vary from person to person, and from time to time with any given person. (D. Williams)

[5]We all have different personalities and our pattern of stuttering is distinct and interwoven in the unique personalities. (Garland)

ingly we ask you to bear with us when you read about troubles which you may not encounter yourself but which may represent a problem to others.

Most have certain abilities which seem somewhat surprising. Nearly all those who stutter generally have little or no difficulty when they sing, shout, whisper, or read in unison with others.[1]

If you have no difficulty talking when you are alone or when you are reading or speaking in unison with others, that would indicate that you have the physical ability to speak normally.

Having the physical ability to speak normally would make it evident that fear or anticipation of trouble or fear may cause you to put unnecessary tension into your speech mechanism and that may trigger most of your difficulty.

In this connection, we would add that this in no way infers that any mental deficiency is involved since it is believed that the I.Q. (intelligence quotient) of the average stutterer is normal or above normal.[2,3,4]

---

[1]Most stutterers have certain abilities which are somewhat surprising. Even the most severe stutterers generally have little or no difficulty when they sing, shout, whisper, speak to a rhythmic stimulus such as a metronome, speak or read in unison with another speaker or speak to a masking noise. (Ramig)

[2]Because you stutter it doesn't mean that you are any more maladjusted than the next person. (Sheehan)

[3]On the whole people who stutter are highly intelligent and capable. (Barbara)

[4]Some famous people who stutter have been of above normal intelligence: Winston Churchill, Charles Darwin, Lewis Carroll, Jack Welch of General Electric, actor James Earl Jones, etc.

Original Cause of Your Stuttering

Many stutterers have mistakenly believed that if only the "cause" could be found, a fast cure would result. Many theories have been advanced to explain the nature and causes of stuttering, but none of them has been proven at this time.

Considerable research is being carried out to investigate possible neurological involvement,[1,2] dominance of one cerebral hemisphere over another, and any factors which may cause a lack of speech muscle coordination resulting in stuttering. Hereditary factors also play a role in some people who stutter.[3]

> "Many have mistakenly believed that if only the 'cause' could be found, a fast cure would result."
> —Murray

Whatever the cause or causes, you need to be concerned about what you are doing now that perpetuates and maintains your difficulty, not about what happened in the past.[4]

There is no reason for you to spend the rest of your life stuttering helplessly. You can gain confidence in your ability to communicate freely.

Others have prevailed, and so can you.

---

[1]Recent evidence from brain imaging studies provides a coherent albeit preliminary view that stuttering occurs when a neurophysiologic system...fails. (Watson)

[2]Any differences between stuttering and non-stuttering speakers involve not only brain regions involved in motor planning and execution, but also those areas important for processing of sensory feedback. (De Nil)

[3]Inheritance clearly plays a role in some cases of stuttering. Ongoing studies of individuals in stuttering families give us important information about the causes of stuttering. (Drayna)

[3]Kang, C., Riazuddin, S., Mundorff, J., Krasnewich, D., Friedman, P., Mullikin, J., and Drayna, D. *Lysosomal Enzyme Targeting Pathway Mutations and Persistent Stutterng.* New England Journal of Medicine Volume 362 pp.677-685 (2010).

[4]Many stutterers have mistakenly believed that if only the "cause" could be found, a fast cure would result. (Murray)

Factors Affecting Therapy

Before explaining the specific steps to be used in therapy, certain relevant factors should be discussed. This is because these factors can affect your attitude toward and your ideas about treatment and how you can and should work on it.

These factors include information on subjects which can have a substantial influence on progress in therapy, factors such as

  1) feelings and emotions,
  2) tension and relaxation,
  3) distractions,
  4) enlisting help from others, and
  5) your determination or motivation.

We will begin by pointing out how feelings and emotions can and frequently do affect the severity of your difficulty.

Your Feelings and Emotions

Stuttering is no simple speech impediment. It is a complicated disorder which has both physical and emotional aspects. To illustrate the latter, the statement can be made that stuttering is largely what the stutterer does trying not to stutter.[1] In other words, stuttering is like an incredible trick you play on yourself. As you tense in reaction to your stuttering and your feelings about stuttering, you are likely to stutter more.

---

[1] In other words, stuttering is what you do trying not to stutter again. (Johnson)

What happens is that you want to stop stuttering so badly that, as a result, you try to force trouble-free speech.[1] And the more you force, the more tension is built up in your speech mechanism and the more trouble you are apt to have. The mechanism of speech is so delicately balanced that the more you try to stop stuttering, the worse you unwittingly make it.

Stuttering affects one emotionally since being a stutterer can be rough. Possibly you may even think it's a disgrace to be a stutterer even though that is not so. As a result, you may have become extremely sensitive about your difficulty.

It is true that the experience of being blocked or not being able to say what you want to say without stuttering can be really frustrating.[2] As a result, under some circumstances you may become so embarrassed and humiliated that you suffer from feelings of helplessness, shame, inferiority, depression and sometimes self-hatred.[3]

Your emotions may generate so much fear and anxiey that they can affect your attitude toward others and life in general.[4,5] Like the tail that wags the dog, stuttering can alter your personality. If you can become desensitized and learn that you do not have to panic when you

---

[1]The stutterer attempts to force the articulation of his words and speaking now becomes a muscular rather than a mental process. (Bluemel)

[2]Fluency is a fair-weather friend that deserts the stutterer when he needs it most. (Sheehan)

[3]Talking was a highly emotional experience which gave me a feeling of helplessness, failure and defeat. (Freund)

[4]The stutterer develops emotional reactions which permeate his very soul, affect his will and upset his mind. (Martin)

[5]The stutterer feels at most times apart and different from others in his society. He feels that although others also have difficulties in life, they can cope with them and live much more easily with their problems. He feels more permanently crippled than others because of the fact that he cannot hide or conceal his speech difficulty, and therefore, he is on the constant target of their embarrassment, ridicule and disapproval. (Barbara)

stutter or anticipate stuttering, then you can begin to change the way you talk; and progress will come more swiftly.

> Positive changes in attitudes and feelings about yourself and your stuttering will lead to positive changes in your speech.

Positive changes in attitudes and feelings about yourself and your stuttering will lead to postive changes in your speech.

Stuttering fears can be of words or sounds, or some persons, of certain situations, of the telephone, of saying your name, of a job interview, etc. When you have little fear, you have less tension and probably will not have as much difficulty.

When your fear is strong, it builds up tension in your speech mechanism and you will stutter more frequently and severely. Sometimes this fear can be so strong as to make you frantic and almost paralyze thought and action.

Such fear or anxiety may prevent you from entering situations and experiences that you would otherwise enjoy. This may cause more shame and embarrassment, and the more frustrated you become, the more you are likely to stutter.

As one person expressed it, "If you can't afford to stutter, you will." So your stuttering is usually in proportion to the amount of fear you have.[1]

Tension and Relaxation

Since fear builds up excessive muscular tension, its reduction should be a major goal of therapy. Tension, gen-

---

[1]The more one stutters, the more he fears certain words and situations. The more he fears the more he stutters. The more he stutters the harder he struggles. The more he struggles, the more penalties he receives, and the greater becomes his fear. (Van Riper)

erated by fear, plays a most important part in activating your stuttering and may be the immediate triggering cause of your difficulty.[1,2,3] If you didn't try to force trouble-free speech, you wouldn't stutter as much or at least you would stutter more easily.

How can tension be reduced? That's difficult to answer. It has been suggested that hypnotism might help. It would be wonderful if you could reduce or eliminate your tension by getting some sort of hypnotic treatment, but unfortunately, hypnosis has not been shown to have any permanent effect.[4]

In an effort to relax, many stutterers have experimented with drinking alcoholic beverages or getting slightly intoxicated. Although this may result in stuttering changes for some people, the effect is only temporary. Obviously, it cannot be recommended.[5,6]

Although there are new drugs, which work to reduce fear and anxiety, unfortunately there are no drugs approved specifically for stuttering at this time.[7,8]

---

[1]Crucial to this point is the fact that struggle and avoidance worsen a problem of stuttering. (Moses)

[2]Stuttering results when the speaker is unable to cope with excess muscular tension in the speech mechanism. (Luper)

[3]Stuttering then may be considered to be in large part something people do when they become unusually tense about the way they talk. (Bloodstein)

[4]Many of you have heard about the wonders of hypnosis and may look to this technique to provide a quick answer. Rest assured that this has been tried throughout the years, but almost invariably with only temporary and fleeting success. (Murray)

[5]I turned to smoking excessively and drinking occasionally but found no solace there. (Wedberg)

[6]One of my patients was a city official who made a practice of taking whisky before giving his weekly report to the City Council. Soon his alcoholism became a more serious problem than his stammering, and he was hospitalized for this condition. (Bluemel)

[7]Since the exacerbation of stuttering by anxiety is a common experience, it might be assumed that drugs that relieve anxiety would be beneficial. (Rosenberger)

[8]Even though medications for stuttering may be on the horizon, no form of therapy for stuttering is a cure. Therefore, future treatment will likely involve the combination of medication with speech therapy to achive the optimal results. (Maguire)

Moreover, in many cases, drugs may bring their own set of side effects to the problem.

It has also been suggested that relaxation exercises help to reduce or eliminate the tension that you experience. It would be good if you could practice relaxation procedures that would eliminate tension and retain their effectiveness during moments of stuttering.

Much research has gone into studying this subject, and many people who stutter have spent thousands of hours trying out such procedures in the hope that their effect would carry over to their time of need. However, the results have not proved satisfactory.[1]

Learning to relax can always benefit your speech, general health, and well-being even if it is not indicated as a solution to the problem. The fundamental principle holds that the more calm and relaxed you are, the less stuttering you will do.[2] That's one reason you will be asked to talk in a smooth, slow, easy and deliberate manner as it will help to induce a calmer and more relaxed way of speaking.

More practical than general relaxation is the relaxation of specific muscles. When you can locate the place where the most tension is, it is possible for you to learn to relax those muscles during speech.[3] This will be particularly helpful.

These exercises involve only certain muscles, the ones you use to control your lips, your tongue, your mouth,

---

[1]Relaxation has sometimes been described as a method in and of itself for the treatment of stuttering. I do not believe, however, that relaxation procedures have much permanent value unless they are part of a more inclusive therapeutic process. (Gregory)

[2]A few minutes of meditation and relaxation each day can help the spirit. (G. Johnson)

[3]Once the stutterer has localized the places in the vocal tract where he habitually exerts too much tension, he may practice stuttering with less of it. (Bloodstein)

your breath and to some extent your vocal cords. When you are relaxed and alone, you can practice purposely tensing and then relaxing those muscles. It will certainly be beneficial if you can relax these muscles during speech.

The regular practice of body exercises is also recommended. The thought is that physical exercises are not only good for one's health but can also contribute to building the self-confidence which all stutterers need.

Body exercises can promote the inclination to stand up straight with head erect and shoulders back.[1] This kind of assertive posture can help generate a feeling of self-confidence - the feeling that you are as good as or better than the next person.[2] In this respect, physical exercises will help you.

Try to adopt a positive attitude generally. Tell yourself that you can and will overcome your difficulty. If you adopt an assertive attitude and combine it with controlled techniques, you will improve faster. Be assertive and believe in yourself and have confidence in your endeavors.[3]

Distractions

If there were some way to distract your mind from thoughts of fear so that you didn't think about your stuttering, you would probably have no trouble.[4] If you could forget you were a stutterer, you might not stutter at all, but

---

[1]Accept the fact that you have a serious problem. Stand squarely on both feet, place your shoulders back and begin to earnestly attack your problem. (Barbara)

[2]Assume an assertive posture - physically be committed to moving forward. Use your body language to advantage. (G.F. Johnson)

[3]This view holds that any human problem is, in many important ways, a disorder of thinking. (Manning)

[4]If he forgot he was a stutterer and simply went ahead on the assumption that he would have no difficulty, he would speak quite normally. (Bloodstein)

we don't know how you could develop such a "forgettery."

Anything that distracts your mind from fear or takes your mind off the anticipation of stuttering will usually give you temporary relief. This is the main rea-

> Distraction...may temporarily blot our thoughts of fear but will not result in any permanent reduction of fear or stuttering.

son why stutterers are sometimes misled by tricky procedures such as talking with sing-song inflection, metronome timing, talking while tapping a finger, swinging an arm, or stamping a foot, etc. These and many other odd ways of talking may produce temporary fluency.

Just thinking about how to use them when you anticipate trouble shifts your attention away from stuttering. They may temporarily blot out thoughts of fear but will not result in any permanent reduction of fear or stuttering.

Strange as it may seem, almost any new or bizarre technique[1,2] will temporarily help any stutterer—at least until the novelty wears off—if he has confidence in its effectiveness.

Enlisting the Support of Others

It would be fortunate if you could find the help of a competent speech-language pathologist trained in the field of stuttering. However, this self-therapy program has been planned under the assumption that you may not

---

[1]One of the tricky features of undertaking therapy with stutterers is that anything in the way of technique to bring about immediate fluency is likely to work at least temporarily. (Sheehan)

[2]Witchcraft, the surgeon's knife, appliances for the tongue, drugs, hypnotism, psychoanalysis, arm swinging and a host of other devices and methods have been employed, and a few 'cures' seem to be obtained by any method, no matter how grotesque. (Van Riper)

have such specialized help. Even if you do, the success of any program is still largely dependent on your efforts.[1,2]

This does not mean that you should discourage help from others as you need people to talk with and practice on. If you have a family member or close friend with whom you have a good and trusting relationship, he or she may be able to render you valuable service in many ways.[3]

Acting as an observer, such a person may be able to see and hear things of which you may not be aware. It is also possible that when you are studying the way you stutter (which will be discussed later), such a friend could duplicate your stuttering to help you become aware of what you are doing when you are having trouble.[4]

Or he or she could accompany you on some of your assignments, compliment you on your efforts, give you moral support by encouraging you to carry on and persevere until you reach your goal. You will need all the encouragement you can get.

Sometimes friends with the best of intentions offer unsolicited advice about what they have heard or think you should do to overcome your stuttering. Although such advice may be unwise and unwanted, we suggest that it should be accepted gracefully even though it is based on an inadequate understanding of the problem.

---

[1]The stutterer must get out of his mind that he can be "cured" by somebody else. (Wedberg)

[2]Before you begin to follow any specific program for correcting your stutter you must remember that stuttering is your problem and yours alone. (Barbara)

[3]What I needed was not an authority but a friend and collaborator genuinely interested in me and ready to help me. I was fortunate to have a brother who could be this friend. (Freund)

[4]My high school chemistry teacher, a former stutterer, gave up his lunch hour twice a week to talk with me about speech...Perhaps you can find this kind of sympathetic friend who will listen while you talk about your stuttering. Let him know that you do not expect advice. You don't expect him to be a clinician, just a friend. (Brown)

26

In some places, support groups of stutterers have been organized. They meet regularly to help each other to work on their problem. If such a group has capable leadership, it can be very worthwhile. *For further information, see* **page 144.**

Your Determination

There is no easy road to fluency. For therapy to accomplish its purpose, it will take determination.[1] It is necessary for you to have the courage to confront[2] your stuttering head-on and undertake assignments

There is no easy road to fluency.

which will require a lot of work and probably a lot of embarrassment.[3] Is more fluent speech worth the effort which you must go through to produce it? That is up to you.

Actually, the embarrassment you experience will help reduce the sensitivity which makes your stuttering worse.[4]

And becoming less sensitive to your difficulty will make it easier for you to retain sufficient presence of mind to carry through on the recommended procedures.

---

[1]You appreciate most in life those things you do for yourself. Getting over stuttering takes tremendous self-discipline and desire. (Aten)

[2]Although it is a tough row to hoe at first, there is nothing as therapeutic as self-confrontation. (Rainey)

[3]Alleviating one's stuttering is ultimately a matter of self-discipline and control. (Stromsta)

[4]At some point in the therapy process the stutterer must become desensitized to his stuttering. (Kamhi)

If you feel your stuttering is a handicap, you need to find ways and means to have a richer life through more fluent speech.[1] You need to feel better about yourself as a person.

Although you should not demand or expect perfection, you want to speak more freely. But to do this, you need the determination to make changes in your way of talking and in yourself. These changes can put you in control and make you master of your speech.

Be assertive and believe in yourself.

We say that you can succeed, and that the pay-off is far greater than the cost. But it will take dedication on your part to change your attitude toward your problem.[2] Stuttering is a stubborn handicap and it will not give up easily.[3,4] Therapy is a challenge.[5] The decision is yours.

---

[1]I still remember vividly what a severe stutterer and how tangled emotionally I once was. When I see any stutterer I remember my own unfavorable prognosis, my own weakness, my lack of hope, and when I do, I find in the case before me strengths and potentials which I did not have. If I could do what I have done, then surely this person could do as much. This is a very real faith, and I suspect it has played a large part in any success I have had as a clinician. (Van Riper)

[2]Leonard, a stutterer, would try anything, although never in a reckless or foolhardy fashion. He possessed both discernment enough to see what needed to be done and guts enough to do it—a happy combination for a stutterer. He had kind of a stubbornness or dogged persistence that he was able to turn into an asset. (Sheehan)

[3]Stuttering is a tough opponent. It never gives up. You've got to keep knocking it down to stay in command. (Starbuck)

[4]A valuable precondition for successful therapy is the deep inner conviction of the stutterer in the creditability of his disorder—combined with a fighting spirit and a readiness to undergo hardships and deprivations. (Freund)

[5]Men who have achieved in this world have been guided by inspiration, by vision, by faith in themselves and by faith in the unknown. (Wedberg)

The Premise and the Program

The ideas expressed in this book are based on the premise that stuttering is a behavior that can be modified or changed. This means that you can learn to control your difficulty, partly through changing your feelings and attitudes about stuttering, and partly through eliminating or correcting the irregular behaviors associated with your stuttering.[1,2,3]

This will involve reducing your fear of having difficulty by disciplining yourself to face your fears and become less sensitive about your stuttering.[4,5] And it will include:

    (1) analyzing your stuttering behavior,
    (2) eliminating unnecessary or abnormal things
        you may be doing, and
    (3) taking positive action to control your blocks.

---

[1]The basic fact revealed by these clinical studies was that stuttering is extremely modifiable. It is possible for a speaker to change drastically the things he does that he calls his stuttering. (Johnson)

[2]During the process of therapy he (the stutterer) should learn by experience that he can change his speaking behavior and that he can change his emotional reactions, both to the way he talks and toward his listeners and himself. (D. Williams)

[3]Basically there are two principal features of his behavior that the stutterer can alter. One is the speech behavior itself and the other is his attitude toward speaking and stuttering in particular. These two aspects are related: one of the ways change of attitude is brought about is by helping the stutterer to experience an ability to modify his speech, and one way in which speech is changed is through the reduction of fear which accompanies a different way of thinking about the problem. (Gregory)

[4]Somehow you must learn to desensitize yourself to the reactions of others and refuse to let people's actual or imagined responses to your stuttering continue to affect your mental health or peace of mind. (Adler)

[5]One of the most important phases of the treatment of the adult stutterer is that which attempts to change the shame and embarrassment that are associated with the act of stuttering. (Van Riper)

The basic principle is that stuttering is something you are doing and you can learn to change what you are doing.[1]

About the Program

Since it is important for you to understand the overall therapy plan, we explain briefly how this program works.

First, you will be asked to try out a helpful therapy procedure described in the next chapter. This will be particularly beneficial for those who feel they need some immediate relief.

Then it is suggested that you comply with twelve common sense helpful recommendations or ground rules to improve your speech. These ground rules are designed to supply you with practical ways of coping with your difficulty.

By complying with the recommendations of these rewarding ground rules, you will be concentrating on reducing both the severity and abnormality of your difficulty and reducing the number of your stutterings. And when you carry out the provisions of these guidelines, you will be gradually laying the groundwork for gaining positive control of your speech.

These rules will urge you to

(1) talk more deliberately,
(2) stutter more easily and openly,
(3) make no effort to hide your stuttering,
(4) stop all avoidance practices,
(5) eliminate your secondary symptoms, and
(6) maintain normal eye contact.

---

[1] Your stuttering is something you do, not something that happens to you. It is your behavior—not a condition. There are mistakes you can correct with a little self-study and courage. (Sheehan)

One particularly important rule will call for you to make a detailed study of what your speech mechanism is doing incorrectly when you stutter. In other words, find out specifically what you are doing when you are having trouble.[1,2]

This essential information will be used to help you change those things you are doing abnormally which make your speech a problem and help you learn better ways of coping with your stuttering.[3]

You should look upon your stuttering as certain things which you have learned to do—not as something which is wrong with you or which happens to you. You should try to substitute normal speech behavior of which you are basically capable for the undesirable ways of reacting which you have learned.

...you must learn to desensitize yourself to the reactions of others...

Then you will be instructed on how to cope with these irregularities by using post-block, in-block and pre-block corrections. These are the technical names of the methods which you will learn in order to help you move smoothly through feared words in a predetermined manner and enable you to develop a feeling of control.

When you find that you can comply with the ground rules, you will have made progress in controlling your

---

[1]The first phase of therapy involves assisting persons who stutter to attend to what they are doing as they stutter. (D. Williams)

[2]You've got to examine and analyze the act of speaking to see what errors you're making. You must be making mistakes somewhere or you would be speaking fluently. What are you doing that makes your speech come out as stuttering? (Starbuck)

[3]For some stutterers simply identifying stutterings as they are being produced is sufficient to enable them to start modifying these very same instances of stuttering. (Conture)

speech. Some rules may affect your stuttering and mean more to you than others because they may hit your weak points. As a result, you will find that attaining the goal of some rules will contribute more to progress in your case.

Unfortunately, there is no way for us to know the particular way you stutter, so we can only suggest that you try to follow through on all the recommendations.

The length of time needed to accomplish the objective of each rule will vary considerably depending on the severity of your case and your resolution in working on the assignments. It is possible that the time required to reach some desired goal can be measured in days.

Even if your stuttering is mild, you are urged to move through each phase of the program.

However, for others, it may take a long time to bring under control some stubborn or seemingly uncontrollable habit.[1,2]

Even if your stuttering is mild, you are urged to move through each phase of the program. And when you tackle a guideline we hope you will feel satisfied that you have reasonably achieved its goal before proceeding to the next one. By doing this, you will know exactly where you stand and what progress you are making.

Learning how to help yourself should be the goal of every stutterer. Your first step will be for you to experiment with a different way of talking as described in the next chapter. This is designed to give you some immediate relief.

---

[1]The adult stutterer enters therapy...the first thing he must understand is that stuttering as it now exists was acquired over a period of time, and that change is a process which will be gradual—not sudden. (Gregory)

[2]But you say you want to stop stuttering. Sure! But first you need to break up the habit pattern that you have built up over the years and this cannot be done instantly. (Emerick)

A Helpful
Therapy Procedure

This procedure is particularly for those stutterers who feel that they need some immediate relief, even if it is temporary. However, it is suggested that you should try out this experimental procedure, since it can help you talk more fluently.

It involves talking in a very slow, smooth prolonged manner. In speaking slowly, it is suggested that you should take as long as a second or more to slide through the beginning or starting sound of all words or syllables.

Then continue to prolong sounds, syllables and words in a smooth, easy onset manner.

...change almost always feels uncomfortable...give yourself time...

This easy onset slow drawn-out method of talking, particularly in starting words, cannot help but give you some relief. It may be particularly helpful to those who do not have many strong negative feelings about their stuttering.

We suggest that you try this procedure. At first, you may not like the way it sounds or feels, but remember that making a change almost always feels uncomfortable. Therefore, we don't recommend talking this way all the time at first. Give yourself time to become accustomed to this new manner of speaking.

See next page for details on how to follow through on this method of treatment.

Specifics

As you are aware, words are made up of sounds. In this procedure, you are asked to start the sounds of your words at an extremely slow, easy, smooth rate by gently and easily sliding extremely slowly through the first sound. This could mean taking as long as a second or more to slide through the beginning sounds that start your words. This is called "easy onset."

Then stretch out and prolong all sounds as you voice them using continuous phonation.[1] That means stretching out and prolonging practically every consonant and vowel sound, and sliding through and slowing the transition from one sound to the next sound.[2]

To do this, start your vocal cords vibrating in a low, steady, very slow way as you begin to make the sounds of your words in this easy onset manner with light pressure in your tongue and lips, also known as "light contacts." You can tell if your vocal cords are vibrating by putting your hand on your throat where you should feel the vibrations.

This extremely slow, drawn-out manner of starting and prolonging all sounds will result in your having continuity of sound and airflow with no break in your voicing and no repetitions. To repeat, stretch out and prolong all your voicing of sounds, particularly the starting sounds. And prolong all transitions between all sounds (consonant and vowel) with light, easy contacts on the consonants.

It is easy to stretch out and prolong vowel sounds, but you will need to practice stretching many of the consonant sounds.[3] Spend time when alone practicing how to

---

[1] Audible sound prolongations are excellent places to start modifications with adult stutterers. (Conture)

[2] What is required to facilitate fluency is to slow the speed of transitional movements from sound to sound which is what prolongation of voice sounds provides. (Perkins)

[3] Achieve the proper slow rate not by pausing between words, but by stretching each vowel and consonant. Vowels are easy to stretch. Consonants are hard. (Guitar-Peters)

increase the duration of consonant sounds as some of them such as t, d, p, b, etc. are "plosive" or "stopping sounds" but need to be spoken easily and slowly with light or loose contacts of the tongue and mouth.

This smooth, slow, easy onset, drawn-out manner of talking should be used on non-feared words as well as feared words. In short, it should be done all the time you talk until you get the knack of it. Bind the sounds of your words together, hitch the beginning of one word to the tail of the preceding one.

You may feel uncomfortable or embarrassed to talk at this easy, smooth, slow rate of only some 30 words per minute, but you need to find out what it can do for you.

To repeat, it is recommended that you use this smooth, prolonged way of talking when speaking to others after you have spent considerable time practicing it when alone.[1]

You may hesitate to talk this way because you feel people will wonder why you are doing so. Tell them the truth - that you are working on your stuttering. There is nothing to be ashamed of, and your friends will be glad to help. After using this manner of talking for some time, one may slowly and gradually increase the rate at which the words are started and spoken, unless trouble occurs. In this case, you should go back to the slower rate at which you had no difficulty.

---

[1]Any action that emphasizes or enhances smooth transitions from sound to sound, syllable to syllable, or word to word, will be beneficial for on-going speech. (Agnello)

This easy onset, slow, flowing manner of talking is a commonly used procedure which can give you considerable relief and enable you to speak more easily. It may not solve your problem completely but will most likely be helpful.

In any event, it will show you and others that you are accepting your stuttering as a problem, not as a curse, and are working to cope with it. People respect that attitude. Start now.

Conscientiously work for some time—possibly a couple of weeks or more on the program as described above. By then you will know what benefit you can derive from this approach to therapy.

Reminder—The quotations and footnotes in this book have been taken from the writings of speech pathologists and medical doctors. They have earned degrees as doctors of philosophy or medicine and know what you are up against as they have been stutterers themselves. They understand your problem from observation and experience and represent a most distinguished array of authority and prestige in the field of stuttering. Their names and titles are listed starting on page 186. Those who have been stutterers are marked with a star by their name.

The All-Important Ground Rules

Adopting Rewarding Habits and Beneficial Practices

We hope that experimenting with the procedure advocated in the last chapter enabled you to communicate more easily with less difficulty. However, we are not recommending that you permanently employ this manner of talking for several reasons. First, it may not work for you at all times in all situations. You may find it difficult to remember to use the fluency shaping techniques when stressed or excited. Secondly, you may not feel comfortable speaking in this way with all listeners.

The rules described in this chapter will explain how to manage your stuttering by putting into effect certain basic remedial practices. These consist of twelve all-important rules which briefly summarize this program. In a general way, they outline how you can manage your difficulty by taking advantage of two approaches.

First, through modifying your feelings and attitudes about your stuttering by decreasing your speech fears and avoidance behaviors.

Second, through modifying the irregular behaviors associated with your stuttering by using certain techniques which will change the form of your stuttering so you can speak without abnormality.

There are twelve of these rules. We wish we could recommend a simpler program, but unfortunately, as has been pointed out, stuttering is a complicated disorder.

Therefore, it is advisable to take advantage of all the approaches available which can work toward solving your problem.

It is suggested that you first read over and carefully study the rules which are described on the following pages. To make progress, it is necessary for you to do your best to comply with **each** of these—working on them one at a time.

It is best to tackle them in the order in which they are listed, although that is a matter of discretion. As listed, the rules are directed first at reducing the sensitivity you may have about your stuttering and stopping all avoidance habits. Then you will concentrate on correcting what you are doing wrong when you stutter.

Toward this latter objective, an important rule will call for you to make a detailed study of what you are doing unnaturally with your speech mechanism as you stutter. Then this information will be employed to enable you to eliminate those things you are doing unnecessarily and correct what you are doing wrong.

To rectify your faulty speech mechanism behaviors, you will be instructed to use post-block, in-block and pre-block corrections. These terms refer to methods designed to help you move smoothly through feared words in a predetermined manner so you can develop a feeling of control.

Working on accomplishing the objectives of these rules will not be easy—in fact, it may be a long drawn-out, worrisome process. Obviously, it will take time and determination not only to work on reducing your fear of difficulty but also to change the pattern of your speaking behavior.

Some rules may reduce the amount of your stuttering and mean more to you than others because they hit your weak points. As a result, you may find that attaining the goal of some rules may contribute to more progress than others. Unfortunately, there is no way for us to know your particular weaknesses so we can only suggest that you follow through on all the recommendations.

Remember, you are your own therapist, and you may have no one to supervise you if you do not follow through on these rules. Perfect compliance is not possible and is not expected, but results are what you want and need.

Working on these beneficial practices and modifying your stuttering should be the key to your making progress.[1] It may be best to work on trying to comply with only one rule at a time. When you feel you have attained the desired results of that assignment, even though it may take a long time, then tackle the next rule.

Schedule practice sessions to coincide with routine daily activities such as meal times, lunch breaks, or going to and from work or school. **Unscheduled practice generally leads to little or no practice.**

Make a real effort to sincerely comply with each of these guidelines to the best of your ability. It will be worthwhile. Give yourself a strong dose of will power and have confidence in your ability to make progress. The following chapters will explain explicitly how to work on achieving the objective of each rule. Here they are—let's go to work on them.

(Some stutterers feel little or no shame and embarrassment about their stuttering. They need not be as concerned about the rules directed at reducing shame and embarrassment as others do.)

---

[1]It is surprising how much just the mentioning and demonstration of these and other corrective techniques can add to your ability to use them and how much they can increase the speaking comfort of both yourself and your listener. (Vinnard)

Therapy must be practiced full time to be highly successful. You must feel that you are on the right track and you must be committed to putting the program into practice. Plan your work well, then work your plan harder than you have ever worked before. Success will follow. (Boehmler)

When you go into therapy, when you begin to modify your speech pattern, go full tilt, reach for the home run...Quit feeling sorry for yourself.

—Emerick

(1) Make a habit of always talking slowly and deliberately whether you stutter or not. It is better to go too slow than too fast.[1] It is easier to control a slow turtle than a fast rabbit, so slow down.

This first guideline calls for you to build the habit of always talking slowly and deliberately. This induces a manner of talking which is generally respected. But it is mainly recommended because it will result in a more varied and relaxed manner of speaking which is more responsive to therapy procedures.[2]

Also, taking your time when talking tends to counteract feelings of time pressure that stutterers sometimes have when called on to speak. Some speak too quickly, trying to get their words out before they stumble or block. This just tends to generate tension and aggravates their stuttering.[3]

To help reduce time pressure, it is also suggested that when you talk, you should often pause momentarily between phrases (or sentences). This will help lessen time-pressure reactions.[4]

Temporarily accepting your role as a stutterer, resolve to make a special effort to talk slowly and deliberately all the time. It may not be easy to do and will take concentration, particularly if you have been in the habit of speaking rapidly. It may also feel unnatural at first, but if you can adjust to this manner of talking, it will be beneficial. Most importantly, you will be under much less time pressure.[5]

*See **page 61** for details on how to follow through on this rule.*

---

[1]Talk slowly and deliberately. (Agnello)

[2]Panic, tension and an overwhelming urgency are the hallmark of stuttering: they are what you need to overcome. (J. D. Williams)

[3]Slowing down the rate of speech has been found to be a strong aid to reducing stuttering. (Stromsta)

[4]Remember speech sounds better in short phrases with frequent pauses. (Aten)

[5]Rate is a particularly useful clinical entry point for establishing fluency and maintaining it. (Perkins)

(2) When you start to talk, do it easily, gently and smoothly without forcing and prolong the first sounds of words you fear. That means talking firmly with your voice smoothly flowing into the sounds of words with light, loose movements of your lips, tongue and jaw.[1]

This most important guideline suggests that when you stutter, slide smoothly and gently into the words in as easy and calm manner as possible.[2] If you can comply with this one rule and let yourself stutter easily, your severity will lessen and so will the frequency of your stuttering.

Also, this rule recommends that while talking easily, you prolong the first sound of any word you fear. And furthermore, that you make a point of prolonging the transition to the next sound or sounds of that word.[3] This only refers to words you fear.

It is not suggested here that you prolong all sounds of all words.

Some try to cope with their problem by trying to force words out at the same time as they close off the airway by squeezing the lips together, or pressing the tongue tightly against the lips together, or pressing the tongue tightly against the roof of the mouth. This makes no sense. You can't pour water out of a corked bottle. Explore how easily you can stutter.

Substitute easier ways of stuttering for your abnormal and frustrating habits.[4] Stutter easily and calmly. You will feel the difference.

*See **page 65** for details on how to follow through on this rule.*

---

[1]Many stutterers have learned as I have learned that it is possible to stutter easily with little struggle and tension. (Sheehan)

[2]Your immediate goal should be to allow yourself to stutter openly and without tension and struggle. (Murray)

[3]Stutterers should be trained in learning how to make slow transitions between the first sound of a feared word and the rest of the word. (Van Riper)

[4]You must learn to substitute easy, slower, more relaxed movements for rushed, tight, forced movements. (Aten)

(3) Stutter openly and do not try to hide the fact that you are a stutterer. Bring it into the open as there is no advantage in pretending that you are a normal speaker.[1,2]

Trying to hide your stuttering only helps to perpetuate it. Tell people with whom you talk that you are a stutterer and adopt an attitude of being willing to stutter voluntarily. If you adopt a frank and open attitude, it will help to reduce what shame and embarrassment you may have about your difficulty.

Feelings of shame and embarrassment only tend to increase your fear of difficulty. And fear of difficulty helps to build up tension or tightness in your speaking apparatus which aggravates your trouble.[3,4,5]

If stutterers did not try to hide the fact that they stutter, most of them would be less sensitive about their problem and, as a result, have much less difficulty. To desensitize yourself and increase your self-confidence is a difficult assignment as it will take time to get rid of your fear. However, the more you work at it, the happier you will be.

Practice openly the techniques you have learned to reduce the frequency and severity of your stuttering blocks. This should add to your ability to use them more easily.

---

[1]The first thing you must become is an honest stutterer. (Starbuck)

[2]Many stutterers will go to any lengths to conceal from others the fact that they stutter. There is great fear of losing face. (Murray)

[3]If you are like all of the other adult stutterers I have known, you create, without meaning to, of course, a major share of any adjustment difficulties you may have...by trying to cover up, conceal or disguise the fact that you talk the way you do. (Johnson)

[4]In order to reduce the amount of stuttering you do, you must reduce your fear of stuttering. (Trotter)

[5]Your fear of stuttering is based largely on your shame and hatred of it. The fear is also based on playing the phony role pretending your stuttering doesn't exist. You can do something about this fear if you have the courage. You can be open about your stuttering above the surface. You can learn to go ahead and speak anyway to go forward in the face of fear. (Sheehan)

Therefore, let's work on reducing the fear you may have about your speech by willingly admitting to others that you are a stutterer. Find occasions to discuss it with those with whom you talk.[1,2] Tell them you are working on your speech.

One objective of this important rule is to increase your ability to tolerate stress and build your self-confidence through desensitization.

As part of this guideline you will be encouraged to sometimes stutter voluntarily on purpose. By deliberately doing what you dread, you may be able to get some relief from the fear and tension which aggravate your problem.

*See **page 69** for details on how to follow through on this rule.*

Yes, I am a stutterer, and I hope that it will help any stutterer who may read this to know that I was such a severe stutterer that I could not put two meaningful words together until I was twenty-four years old. Do I still stutter? Oh, I call myself a stutterer because I still have small interruptions in my speech now and then. But, there's another more important reason why I call myself a stutterer. I'm not trying to hide the fact anymore!

—Rainey

----

[1]They should cultivate the ability to discuss their stuttering casually and objectively with others. (Bloodstein)

[2]You need to communicate more openly and easily with other people including being frank about your stuttering. (Boland)

(4) Identify and eliminate any unusual gestures, facial contortions, or body movements which possibly you may exhibit when stuttering or trying to avoid difficulty.

This does not refer to what you do incorrectly with your muscles of speech which will be carefully investigated later. The above rule refers to unnecessary mannerisms or noticeable movements which may characterize the particular pattern of the way you stutter; these are called "secondary symptoms."

Secondary symptoms include such things as head jerks, eye blinking or closings, hand or arm movements, foot tapping, ear pulling, knee slapping, raising eyebrows, facial grimaces, finger tapping, covering your mouth with your hand, etc., etc.

To accomplish this, it will be necessary to find out and identify what secondary symptoms you have. This information is needed so you can work at eliminating them. These are bad habits which possibly you may have fallen into, thinking they would help you speak more easily but in fact they only add to the abnormality of your stuttering.[1]

Possibly you have no such unnatural behaviors, but check yourself carefully as described in the chapter on eliminating secondary symptoms.[2] If you find you have such behaviors, let's work on getting rid of them. Obviously, they are not necessary for the production of speech.[3]

*See **page 77** for details on how to follow through on this rule.*

---

[1]When these reactions are recognized as secondary symptoms, they can gradually be minimized and controlled and the stammerer is then in a better position to contend with the primary speech disorder. (Bluemel)

[2]Become aware of head or arm movements, eye blinking, other movements or body rigidity, lip smacking or other noises, puffing of the cheeks or pressing the lips. (Moses)

[3]He (the stutterer) will learn, much to his surprise, that these secondary symptoms are not an integral part of his disorder, that it is possible for him to stutter without using them. (Van Riper)

(5) Do your best to stop all avoidance, postponement or substitution habits which you may have acquired to put off, hide or minimize your stuttering. It is very important to make a practice of not avoiding, postponing or substituting.[1]

Much of a your difficulty may be traced to avoidance practices. While temporarily affording relief, such habits actually increase your fears and cause more trouble in the long run.[2] For instance, if the telephone rings and you refuse to answer because you are afraid you won't be able to talk well, the act of avoiding this situation will only tend to build up your fear of the telephone.[3]

To help cancel fear, you should do your best to not dodge speaking situations, avoid social contacts, give up speech attempts or leave the scene of approaching trouble, substitute words or use postponements.[4] Don't avoid words you might stutter on—and keep your appointments.

This can be a really tough assignment but many authorities feel that non-avoidance will give you more relief than any other therapy procedure.[5] Avoidances have been described as a pump in the reservoir of fear.

---

[1]Don't avoid certain words or situations that trigger stuttering. Face them head-on. It's far better to stutter than to avoid speaking situations because the fear of stuttering just compounds the problem. (Murray)

[2]And what actually happens is that the more you cover up and try to avoid stuttering the more you will stutter. (Barbara)

[3]Avoidance can be defined as a process of shying away from the responsibility of facing your problems. (La Porte)

[4]You must sharply reduce or eliminate the avoidances you use. Everytime you substitute one word for another, use a sound or some trick to get speech started, postpone or give up an attempt at talking, you make it harder for yourself. (Emerick)

[5]The more you run away from your stuttering, the more you will stutter. The more you are open and courageous, the more you will develop solid fluency. (Sheehan)

It would be good if you could develop a feeling inside yourself that you will eagerly hunt out and eliminate avoidances.[1,2] This feeling will come if you can make a practice of doing things you fear without giving yourself time to talk yourself out of them. It is particularly important for the stutterer to establish speech that is avoidance-free.[3]

See **page 85** *for details on how to follow through on this rule.*

Much of your difficulty may be traced to avoidance practices.

---

[1]The stutterer should develop a conscience which itself will penalize the tendency to avoid. (Van Riper)

[2]One of the primary concerns of therapy is to develop in stutterers a conscience that prevents them from avoiding stuttering. (Bloodstein)

[3]Stuttering is one thing that gets a lot easier if you don't try to hide it. (Guitar)

(6) Maintain eye contact with the person to whom you talk. Possibly you may already do so, but if not, start looking your listener in the eye more or less continuously in a natural way.[1] It is particularly important for you not to look away when you stutter or expect to.

Possibly because they are ashamed of their speech difficulty, many who stutter have a tendency to avoid looking at their listener when stuttering.[2,3] Using continuous normal eye contact will work toward reducing feelings of shame and embarrassment. If you do not already maintain healthy, normal eye contact, concentrate on doing so.[4]

*See **page 95** for details on how to follow through on this rule.*

---

[1]Establish eye contact before you begin to speak. Two or three seconds of quiet eye contact can get you off to a better start. (Sheehan)

[2]Try to maintain eye contact with your listeners. Looking away severs the communication link with your audience and convinces them that you are ashamed and disgusted with the way you talk. (Moses)

[3]As a matter of fact I had to tell him that I would feel more comfortable if he would look at me while we talked, and it was interesting that as he began to look at me, he struggled less and less. (Rainey)

[4]Maintaining eye contact may sound easy. For many people it is very hard. I know stutterers who have gone through various therapies with some success but who still have been unable to break their old habit of looking away from their listener when a block begins. (Murray)

(7) Analyze and identify what your speech muscles are doing improperly when you stutter. It is an essential and very important part of this program for you to be able to determine specifically what you are having your speech muscles do incorrectly when you stutter.[1]

This involves finding out what you are doing wrong or unnecessarily which needs to be modified or corrected.[2] To repeat, since you are using your speech muscles improperly when you stutter, it is important for you to discover what you are having them do incorrectly so you can work on correcting them.[3,4]

Making use of such an investigation is a key point in therapy. We urge you to follow through on this rule and study your speech muscle behavior. Then you can duplicate it in order to compare it with your speech when you talk without difficulty.[5,6]

There are various ways to observe yourself. One way would be to hold on to your stuttering blocks long enough to determine what you are doing or stutter slowly enough to give you time to get the feel of what is happening. Or watch yourself in the mirror when making phone calls—or listen to a playback of a tape recording of your speech, etc.

---

[1]When a problem exists, the first thing to do is to examine it carefully with the hope of discovering what is wrong. (Rainey)

[2]Try to identify what you are doing wrong when you stutter. (Emerick)

[3]Another important goal in your search for an ultimate cure is to acquaint yourself with your stuttering behavior. (Barbara)

[4]Pay enough attention to the things you do that interfere with your normal speech, the things you do that you call your stuttering; that is, to understand that they are unnecessary and to change or eliminate them. (Johnson)

[5]For some stutterers simply identifying stutterings as they are being produced is sufficient to enable them to start modifying these very same instances of stuttering. (Conture)

[6]Stutterers need to learn what to do when they do stutter if they are to eventually reduce the fear and frustration involved. (Czuchna)

It is most worthwhile to have videos made of yourself when stuttering. Being able to study what you are doing is a powerful tool in enabling you to work on changing what you are doing wrong. Seeing yourself and hearing yourself stuttering can be both revealing and motivating.

It will take courage to do these things but you definitely want this information to help solve your problem so you will become fully aware of what needs to be modified or corrected.[1] Hopefully you will be able to feel, watch and hear yourself stuttering.[2] With this information it will be possible for you to answer the following three questions:

1) what am I doing?
2) why am I doing it?
3) what else can I do?

Important

See the chapters starting on **page 99** *on finding out what you do when you stutter—and on analyzing blocks. They include a section explaining how one stutterer could work on saying his name without difficulty.*

---

[1]The stutterer must come to know just what he does when he approaches a feared word or situation. (Van Riper)

[2]You, as a stutterer, must study your speech pattern in order to become aware of the differences between stuttered and fluent speech. (Neely)

(8) Take advantage of block correction procedures designed to modify or eliminate your abnormal speech muscle stuttering behavior.

Understanding and efficiently operating these procedures can be the key to your making substantial progress.

These useful procedures include (1) a post-block correction which explains what you should do about a stuttering block after it has occurred, (2) an in-block correction which explains what you should do about a block as it is occurring, and (3) a pre-block correction which calls for you to plan and prepare for it so it will not occur.

They are employed to help you develop a feeling of control by taking advantage of the knowledge gained from the study of your blocking difficulties as discussed under Rule (7).

These are to be put to work only after you have studied and identified what you are doing abnormally with your speech mechanism when you stutter.[1] With the use of this information the block corrections referred to above will help you use the strategy needed to eliminate, modify or correct these abnormalities.[2,3,4]

To follow through on these most significant and important procedures, see chapters on **block corrections** *starting on* **page 113.**

---

[1]You don't have a choice as to whether you stutter but you do have a choice as to how you stutter. (Sheehan)

[2]Stuttering consists mainly of learned behavior. This behavior can be unlearned. (Murray)

[3]Stuttered forms of speech can be changed in various ways just as handwriting can be modified. It is this changing of an established habit that requires work. (Neely)

[4]After the stutterer gains the knowledge of how he stutters through block analysis, he is ready to attack and defeat his most dreaded enemy. This is accomplished by the use of post-block, in-block and pre-block corrections. (Starbuck)

(9) Always keep moving forward as you speak, unless you repeat purposely to emphasize a word or thought. If you stutter, plan to stutter forward so as not to hold or repeat any sound. Some stutterers have the habit of **repeating** sounds which are difficult for them when trying to get through a word (b-b-b-boy, etc.)

When you start and voice a sound or word, there is no use holding or making it over again.[1] Continuing the flow of your voice will work against any tendency to hold a block, prolong or repeat sounds or words on which trouble is anticipated.[2]

The idea is to keep your voice moving forward from one word or sound until the next. When you anticipate trouble on a word, plan to use a prolonged easy onset on the first sound and on the transition to the next sound but keep the voice going forward.[3]

...going back will never get you anywhere worthwhile.

In other words, try to say what you have to say without repeating or back-tracking. Going back to get a running start may possibly get you past a block but will never get you anywhere worthwhile. So do your best not to ever repeat or hold sounds, words or anything unless you are repeating purposely to emphasize a word or thought.

You may not realize what you are doing until you hear and see yourself on tape.

---

[1] Why continue to make a sound when you have already produced it? (Van Riper)

[2] The stutterer needs to stutter forward. He needs to go ahead...without regard to anticipated difficulty. (Sheehan)

[3] Keep going forward slowly but positively. (J. D. Williams)

(10) Try to talk with inflection and melody in a firm voice without sounding affected or artificial. Avoid talking in a monotone and keep varying your speaking rate and its loudness. Speak in a melodious manner without sounding artificial. Using natural expression with variations in tone and rate will make your talking more relaxing and pleasant.

(11) Pay attention to the fluent speech you have. Feel its movements and postures. Don't just be aware of your stuttering. Listen to yourself when you are fluent.[1,2] You need to recognize and remember your successful and pleasant speaking experiences. *Mentally replay successful speaking situations* and feel your fluency to build your confidence.

Remind yourself that you have the ability to speak fluently. To help give yourself that feeling, spend time speaking or reading to yourself when relaxed and alone. Do some of this while watching yourself in the mirror. As you do it, be conscious of the fact that it is possible for you to speak easily without effort in a normal way without difficulty.

---

[1] Pay more attention to your normal speech than to what you think of as you're stuttering. (Johnson)

[2] Practice monitoring your speech while speaking slightly more slowly and deliberately, even when you are perfectly fluent. (Ramig)

(12) While working on this program **try to talk as much as you can** since you will need every opportunity to work on the procedures recommended. This does not mean that you should make a nuisance of yourself but talk more—you've probably been silent long enough. Speak out when you want to.[1,2,3] If opportunities to talk do not exist, you should do your best to create them. Let others hear your ideas. If you can't find a listener, there's always the phone. Call a department store and ask a question.

These are the all-important ground rules which should govern your speech behavior. They briefly outline the practices which should enable you to manage your disorder.

Later chapters in this book will give a more complete description of how to go about complying with these rules. So it is strongly suggested you read and study each chapter identified with each rule.

---

[1]Findings suggest that the more a stutterer talks, the better, and the more people he talks to and the more situations he talks in, the better. (Johnson)

[2]The stutterer should be encouraged to talk as much as possible. (Brown)

[3]Saturate yourself with speech. There is a direct correlation between speaking time and fluency. (G. F. Johnson)

Goals and Challenges

Working on modifying or changing your stuttering is challenging—you will be conquering situations from which you have always retreated.

Focus on the fact that you can change what you are doing, and stuttering is something you are **doing** and not something that happens to you.[1,2]

As you change your speaking behavior, you will find that your emotional reactions will change. When this happens, in turn it will be easier to change your speaking behavior.

Develop a Hierarchy

Let's tackle the problem. How do you go about achieving these goals? Plan to go at it easily but in an organized way with determination.

You may want to start by systematically tackling one rule at a time. Possibly work on one which would be easy and then take the next hardest.

Develop a hierarchy of situations and assignments. That is to say, begin by going from the easiest situation and work your way up. In this way, you gain confidence as you move ahead.[3]

---

[1]Stuttering is a series of activities you do. (Emerick)

[2]Speech is something produced by the speaker and as such is something the speaker can modify and change. (Conture)

[3]Another philosophy of my therapy has been that by tackling situations of increasing difficulty, others that were once hard become easier. (Gregory)

Make a list of 5 to 10 speaking situations going from the easiest to the hardest. Use Ground Rule Number 1, speaking slowly and deliberately, in these situations:

1. talking when alone or with a pet (easiest)
2. talking with a close friend
3. ordering in a restaurant
4. making a phone call to a friend
5. making a phone call to a stranger
6. having a conversation at work
7. participating in a meeting at work (hardest)

You will need to develop your own hierarchy as the points listed here may not be right for you.

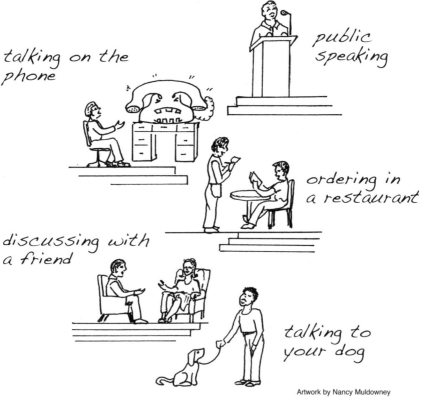

Artwork by Nancy Muldowney

A hierarchy going from easier situations to harder ones.

Set Up a Daily Quota

Set up a daily quota for yourself. You may want to repeat step one—talking with a close friend using Rule One, speaking slowly and deliberately—for several days or even weeks before you move to step two, ordering in a restaurant, speaking slowly and deliberately.

On the first day, collect at least one instance in which you fulfill the requirements of one rule; then two in a row; then three in a row and so on.

Make careful note of your accomplishments in your workbook every day, perhaps in the evening at bedtime. The key is to do it regularly every day more or less at the same time.[1]

Minimum and Maximum Goals

In defining your goals, set up a minimum you feel sure you can do and a maximum that may strain your motivation and yet be achieved. For example, devise the following for the rule calling for you to speak slowly and deliberately. For a minimum goal "I will talk slowly and deliberately while reading aloud to myself for five minutes;" for a maximum goal "I will use it on several phone calls whether I stutter or not." Each day record your performance honestly, and try to cover all of the rules and in subsequent days gradually increase your quota.

---

[1]Adult stutterers have taken many years to develop their speech problem and their reactions to and emotions regarding it. This type of behavioral-emotional complex will not be changed overnight, and we believe the stutterer should be prepared for moments, hours and days of difficulty. We said prepared, and not excused. (Conture)

SAMPLE CHART

	Minimum Goal	Maximum Goal	Results How did I do?
Monday			
Tuesday			
Wednesday			
Thursday			
Friday			
Saturday			
Sunday			

Rewards

It will help if you set up a system to reward yourself. Find something you'd like to do such as reading a magazine for an hour, watching TV or eating a snack, etc., and let yourself do it only after you have accomplished a specific goal. Alternately, you might allow yourself to buy something you really need or want after you have done so many assignments.

It may be quite difficult for you to comply with some of these guidelines since you are changing habits which you have had for years.[1] If sometimes you try and fail on some of them, do not get disheartened. Others have met difficulties and conquered them. Give it time. If you can only reduce the tension and severity of your struggle behavior by learning to stutter easily and openly, you will have made a lot of progress toward your goal.

The following chapters will discuss most of the recommended procedures and how they can have an impact on your stuttering and the ease with which you speak.

Desirable Equipment

For use in modifying your stuttering habits certain items can be of assistance. One is a reasonably large mirror (at least 15″×18″) which can be moved around and situated where you can observe yourself closely when talking on the phone.

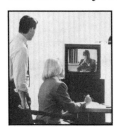

It is important for you to also have on hand a notebook in which to keep records of your work every day.

Also, it will be helpful if you can obtain the use of a voice recorder which you can carry around with you to record the way

---

[1]Listening to yourself stutter on a tape recorder is another good way of helping reduce your fear of stuttering. (Trotter)

you stutter.[1,2] Small recorders not much bigger than your hand are readily available, and they can be purchased at a fairly reasonable price.[3,4] You may not realize what you are doing when you stutter and will only realize it if you hear yourself on tape.

If you can afford the expense, it would be even more advantageous for you to use a video recorder. With its use, you can make videos of your speech. This enables you to both see and hear yourself as you try to speak, just as if you were on television.

If you do obtain a tape recorder, the question will arise as to what is the best way to get recordings. We hope you can find a way. If you have trouble talking on the phone, you might put the recorder nearby when you are making phone calls. Some stutterers have experimented with going into stores to discuss buying items of interest and making recordings of the conversations. At least five or ten minutes of recording time is desirable.

The playback of such recordings can help you identify what you are doing incorrectly.[1,2,3] Any and all recordings should help, and it is important for you to continually make daily notes in your notebook concerning your efforts to make progress.

The following chapters will discuss most of these ground rules and how they can have an impact on your stuttering and the ease with which you can speak.

---

[1]There is nothing like being able to hear your own speech in order to judge what you do and don't like about it and to decide what changes to make as you practice. (J. D. Williams)

[2]By using a tape recorder you tend to learn faster than your stuttering is, indeed, your own doing, and the changes you can make in what you do are very substantial. (Johnson)

[3]A recorder and a mirror are useful in enabling the individual to understand his audible and visible defects of speech. (Ansberry)

[4]A tape recorder will prove a good investment for the stammerer. (Bluemel)

Talking Slowly and Deliberately

The first rule calls for you to build a habit of talking slowly and deliberately, whether or not you stutter. This is recommended for a couple of reasons. First, it induces a manner of talking which is generally respected and admired, and secondly, it will result in a more varied, relaxed manner of speaking which is more responsive to therapy controlled procedures.

Temporarily accepting your role as a stutterer, resolve to make a special effort to talk slowly and deliberately all the time.[1] This will not be easy to do if you normally speak fairly rapidly. It may take considerable effort to talk slowly whenever you speak.

It will help if you can spend at least five to ten minutes a day practicing when you are alone. You might read to yourself at a gradual slow rate in line with what you should use in conversation with others. Then possibly think of some subject about which you are informed and talk to yourself slowly and deliberately.

When you are with others, always try to resist feelings of time pressure. At the moment you are expected to speak, you may sometimes have an almost panicky feeling of haste and urgency.[2,3] You think that you are under "time pressure" with no time to lose, and you have a compulsive feeling that

---

[1] Try stuttering slowly. Keep stuttering, but do it in slow motion. (Guitar)

[2] I have always felt a great pressure to give a reply within a split second and with just the right and exact words. Other stutterers feel this, too. Isn't it silly? (Garland)

[3] Stutterers generally stutter too fast and get into tremors because they do. (Van Riper)

you must speak quickly without taking the time for deliberate and relaxed expression. Do your best to resist this time pressure feeling.[1,2]

Stutterers are also apt to fear silence when they are embarrassed. Accordingly, it is suggested that when talking, you should experiment with occasionally pausing. When speaking a sentence, pause momentarily (very briefly) between words and between phrases. There is no hurry—probably you are not taking as much time as you think—take your time. Unless there is a fire, people will wait to hear what you have to say. Let them wait and don't hurry saying "hello" on the phone. Pause! Take your time.

If you have a tape recorder available, this is an opportune time to make a recording of the way you talk, particularly if you have not yet started speaking according to the recommendations of this first rule.

Making a recording of the way you usually stutter will supply important information to be used in this program.[3] For example, listening to such a recording should help you discover what, if anything, needs to be done to qualify you as speaking slowly and deliberately.

The question arises as to what may be the best way to get a recording of your stuttering. If you have trouble talking on the phone, you might place a microphone near when you make several phone calls—at least five or possibly ten minutes of recording time is desirable.

---

[1]Panic, tension, and an overwhelming urgency are the hallmarks of stuttering; they are what you must overcome. Totally resist any feelings of hurry and pressure. Let 'em wait. (J. D. Williams)

[2]A basic feature of stuttering behavior is that the stutterer is under time pressure to a great extent. The stutterer has to learn how to permit pauses in his speech, to risk the fear of silence, to give himself time to catch his breath to resist the time pressure. (Sheehan)

[3]A tape recorder will prove a good investment for the stutterer. (Bluemel)

Then later, take the time to listen to the recordings. Did you talk slowly and deliberately and thus set an example of the rate at which you should speak? Later you will use these recordings to study your speech.

Of course if possible, it would be even more advantageous in studying your speech if you could have videotapes made of the way you talk. This enables you to both see and hear yourself at the same time.

―――――――――

As a speech pathologist working with adult stutterers, I have found that the most important factors that determine progress are (1) that the stutterer have a goal that requires better speech, and (2) that he form the habit of working consistently and steadily to accomplish his purpose.

—Gregory

―――――――――

When you become aware that the struggling behavior you call stuttering is something you are doing as you talk and not something that magically "happens to you," you are in a very good position to begin to change what you are doing as you talk so you can talk more easily.

—D. Williams

Stuttering Easily
with Prolongation of Feared Words

This most essential second rule suggests that you make a practice of stuttering easily and smoothly without forcing. It doesn't call for you to stop stuttering, but to do it calmly, smoothly, sliding into the sounds of words with light, loose movements of your tongue, lips and jaw.[1] Making light contacts of your speech muscles is sometimes referred to as 'easy onset.'

There is nothing to be gained by trying to force trouble-free speech.[2] Instead, try to maintain an easy, relaxed manner with reduced tension.

Don't struggle when you talk. One of the ways you can tell if you are struggling is to monitor the amount of air pressure in your mouth. Try not to let it build up behind your lips or tongue. Try stuttering with the lips

> Don't try to force trouble-free speech.

loose and the tongue not pressing tightly against your gums or palate. Why erect a blockade in your mouth behind which the air pressure increases greatly?

Most stuttering, to some extent, results from efforts to force trouble-free speech.[3] Unfortunately, the mechanism of speech is too complicated to function properly when force is

---

[1]They (referring to stutterers) must learn to move easily through words rather than recoiling from them. (Czuchna)

[2]We struggle against ourselves trying to force speech. (Garland)

[3]It is in fact probably impossible to stutter in any way at all without excessive muscular tension in some form. (Bloodstein)

applied. So, if you can comply with this rule and let yourself stutter easily, your severity will be lessened and so will the frequency of your stuttering.

Although this may be difficult to carry out, we also recommend that when you are alone, you practice relaxation of your speech muscles. This calls for you to purposely tense yourself, particularly in the mouth area. And then release or reduce the tension so the difference can be felt.

It will also help you talk more easily if you make a point of prolonging the first sound of any word you fear and then prolong the transition to the next sound or sounds of that same feared word.[1]

This does not call for you to prolong all sounds of all words even though possibly you found out in the procedure described on page 33 that it helped you to do this. However, as stated above, it is suggested here that *just on feared words,* you prolong the first sound of such words and then prolong the transition to the next sound or sounds of the same feared words.[2] This could mean taking as long as a second or more in making the gradual transition to the next sound.

Obviously, there are some feared consonant sounds which cannot be prolonged. These consonant sounds are called plosives, referring to the sounds of consonants like 'p,' 'b,' 't,' 'd,' 'k,' etc. Still, with light contacts, you should ease into such sounds by stretching out the following sounds of that word. For instance, on the word 'cat,' make a light contact on the 'k' sound and then make a point of slowly shifting into the vowel sound of the 'a'.

---

[1] By deliberately permitting yourself to prolong the initial sounds of many of the words you will be taking the psychological offensive. (Murray)

[2] Stutterers should be trained in learning how to make slow transitions between the first sound of a feared word and the rest of the word. (Van Riper)

Practice talking smoothly and easily by reading aloud when alone for five to ten minutes a day. Read in a firm voice but keep your speech movements loose and relaxed.[1] The idea is to get accustomed to using gentle, light control of your muscles of speech whether or not you stutter.

Then, of course, it is advisable for you to practice making prolongations of the first sounds of feared words. Probably you have no fear of difficulty while reading alone. Still, while reading you might pick out certain words on which you normally stutter. Then when you come to these words, experiment by slowly shifting into and prolonging the starting sound and then make a particular point of prolonging the transition to the next sound.

It can be a problem to accustom yourself to this easy manner of talking. You will forget at times, but you should use reminders. For instance, you could put up a sign on your clock or mirror reading "remember to easy-stutter today," or put a rubber band on your wrist so you will be continually reminded to direct your efforts toward talking easily while prolonging certain sounds of feared words. You could also make a list at night of the times during the day when you did or did not remember to talk as suggested.

When you are working on these rules, it is well to make a record of your progress in your workbook. First, try for one successful performance, then two in a row, three in a row, etc. until you have been able to collect five consecutive listeners to whom you have spoken slowly in an easy, smooth manner, whether or not you stutter.[2]

---

[1] Feel the relaxed easy movements into and out of words. (Aten)

[2] Most clinicians learn that things work out better if goal-setting is structured in times of maximum and minimum goals. The maximum goal should tax the stutterer's resources or strength to the limit and yet be possible of attainment, while the minimum goal should almost certainly be expected to be achieved. (Van Riper)

We hope you will be able to accustom yourself to effortless talking with prolongation of certain first sounds and transitions. This guideline by itself will not stop your stuttering, but it will help you to be under less tension and stress which will make you happier about your speech.

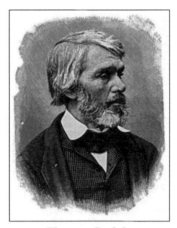

Thomas Carlyle

You might be interested in a quotation by a non-stutterer from a letter written many years ago by Thomas Carlyle, the historian, to Ralph Waldo Emerson, dated November 17, 1843. He said "a stammering man is never a worthless one...It is an excess of delicacy, excess of sensibility to the presence of his fellow-creature, that makes his stammer." Even in those days they realized that sensitivity was an important factor in actuating and maintaining stuttering.

Rule (3)   *(page 43)*

Admitting That You Stutter

The third therapy guideline calls for you to adopt an attitude of being willing to openly admit and not hide the fact that you are a stutterer.[1] You may ask why you should do that when you are trying to not be one.

In order to make headway, it is advisable that you first adopt an attitude of being willing to talk frankly to others about your problem. By doing so, you will be lessening the fear of difficulty you have when talking.

As has been explained, if you are like most stutterers, you are ashamed of the fact that you stutter. As a result you try to keep others from finding out that you are a stutterer. This feeling of shame tends to build up a fear of having difficulty when you are called on to speak at certain times and under certain circumstances.[2]

This fear of difficulty usually builds up tension or tightness in your speech organs which aggravates your trouble. Unfortunately, one's speaking apparatus operates in such a delicate, complex and complicated manner that it is most difficult for it to operate under tension. So the frequency and severity of your difficulty is usually in proportion to the amount of fear and tension you have.[3]

---

[1]You will remain a stutterer as long as you continue to pretend not to be one. (Sheehan)

[2]Stuttering is one thing that gets a lot easier if you don't try to hide it. (Guitar)

[3]It is surprising how much just the mentioning and demonstration of these and other corrective techniques can add to your ability to use them and how much they can increase the speaking comfort of both yourself and your listener. (Vinnard)

To combat fear and tension—your worst enemies[1]—it is necessary to torpedo a lot of your shame and sensitivity. The amount of energy a stutterer may spend in hiding his disorder can be tremendous. Some devise intricate strategies of avoidance and disguise or may even assume some kind of masquerade in the hope, usually a vain one, that the listener won't recognize them as a stutterer. This burden just makes communication more difficult.[2]

Where does all that anxiety and worry get you? Nowhere. It only makes matters worse since it just builds up more fear and tension. So what can or should be done about it? Even if you are not obsessed with hiding the fact that you stutter, it will be helpful to get rid of what worry you do have on this point.

The answer is simple but not easy. You can counteract a lot of that worry and concern by just telling people that you are a stutterer and stop pretending that you are a normal speaker. You should not shirk this assignment. Make occasions to freely admit to those with whom you associate and with whom you normally talk that you are a stutterer and be willing to discuss it with anyone.[3,4,5]

This will take courage on your part, but it needs to be done to reduce your sensitivity.[6] Changing the mental approach toward your problem cannot be done easily and quickly, but the more you work at it, the more you can accomplish. It will pay off to do so. It is no disgrace to be a

---

[1]Many stutterers learn that their greatest enemies are fear and tension. (Aten)

[2]No problem is solved by denying its existence. (Brown)

[3]Whenever you have an opportunity to discuss your stuttering with someone, do it! (La Porte)

[4]This involves telling friends and colleagues that you are a stutterer working on your speech. (Guitar-Peters)

[5]Stutterers must freely admit their problem to associates who may not be aware of it. (Bloodstein)

[6]At some point in the therapy process the stutterer must become desensitized to his stuttering. (Kamhi)

stutterer anyway. You may think so, but you are wrong if you do. Please don't allow your feelings to defeat your efforts.

Start on this assignment by talking with people you are close to and then later with strangers with whom you have conversation. As one person expressed it, "I'm letting the cat out of the bag right away. I'm telling him I'm a stutterer. I used to try to hide this because my greatest fear was having to reveal myself when I met someone. This way, I take the fear out of the situation right away."

Another remarked "It took me twenty years before I would admit to myself, or anyone, that I stuttered. I didn't want to acknowledge that I was different. Yet that is precisely what I needed to do in order to take the first step toward forging a new and more fulfilling identity."

For example, you might say to a friend something to the effect that "you know that I am a stutterer and frankly I have been ashamed to admit it. I need to be more open about my problem and may need your help." Any real friend will appreciate your frankness and will feel closer to you as a result. Besides you will find that people are interested in stuttering. Teach them about it.

Complying with this assignment will reduce your tension, and it will help you accept your stuttering as a problem with which you can cope with less shame and embarrassment.[1] This can make a world of difference and enable you to adopt a more healthy, wholesome and objective attitude toward your difficulty, something all stutterers need so badly.

You may think it will hurt your pride to frankly tell people that you are a stutterer, but it is more likely that you

---

[1]When you begin to really accept yourself as the stutterer you are, you are on your way to much easier speech and most certainly to greater peace of mind. (Rainey)

will be proud of yourself for doing it. Besides there is no use spending your life pretending.[1]

Of course you can't accomplish this goal in a day or two. It will take time to make contact with people you know and carry out this recommendation. No matter how long it takes, it will help reduce your tension and fear if you cultivate an attitude of being willing to talk about your stuttering.[1]

Can you do so? As the fellow said "it ain't easy"—and that's putting it mildly. But this is a most beneficial step toward relieving you of much of your fear and tension.

Voluntary Stuttering

When working on this third rule, it is suggested that you be willing to try experimenting with stuttering voluntarily. Stutterers can usually get some relief from fear and tension by doing this. If you deliberately stutter, you are directly attacking the tension which is aggravating your problem by voluntarily doing that which you dread.[2]

Voluntary stuttering, sometimes called fake or pseudo stuttering, should take the form of easy, simple repetitions or short prolongations of the first sound or syllable of a word or the word itself. It should only be done on **non-feared** words in a calm and relaxed manner.

Do not imitate your own pattern of stuttering but stutter smoothly and easily in a different way.[3,4] Later you will be

---

[1]Your fear of stuttering is based largely on your shame and hatred of it. The fear is also based on playing the phony role of pretending your stuttering doesn't exist. (Sheehan)

[2]When the stutterer does voluntary stuttering, he can say to himself, "I am doing the thing I fear. Also I realize that I can change my speech; I can tell my speech mechanism what to do." (Gregory)

[3]Deliberately stutter! Yes, stutter on purpose in as many situations as possible, but stutter in a different way. (La Porte)

[4]Even if he feels beforehand that he can speak without stuttering, the stutterer is encouraged to pretend or fake stuttering—but to do so in a way different from his usual manner of stuttering. (Barbara)

asked to study and learn about your own pattern, but it is better to stutter in an easy and relaxed way when doing it purposely.

Whatever type of easy stuttering you decide to use, you must be sure to keep it entirely voluntary. It is not advisable to let it get out of control and become involuntary.

Learn to control the uncontrollable.

Experiment by talking slowly and deliberately with easy repetitions or prolongations that differ from your usual pattern. It will give you a sense of self-mastery when you can control the uncontrollable.

Start when alone by reading aloud and calmly, making easy repetitions or prolongations. Then later, work it into conversations with others. Make up assignments for yourself in which you are required to stutter voluntarily.[1] For instance, go into a store and ask the clerk the cost of different items, faking blocks on some words. Make the blocks easy but obvious. Maintain good eye contact while stuttering and be sure to purposely stutter only on words you do not fear.

Voluntary stuttering can help eliminate some of your shame and embarrassment.[2] The more you can follow through and practice doing this, the easier it will become.

---

[1] One means of satisfying the fear of stuttering is to stutter voluntarily on nonfeared words in all kinds of situations. This has the effect of helping you reduce the pressure that you feel when you try to avoid stuttering, and of enabling you to handle your speech more effectively. (Sheehan)

[2] We took Patricia out into a variety of public situations and demonstrated that we could fake stuttering without becoming upset. Gradually she was able to do this herself, first with us along, and then alone…. In this part of the treatment we saw significant changes in Patricia's attitudes. She seemed to be seeking out stuttering instead of avoiding it. (Guitar-Peters)

Aim toward the goal of being willing to stutter without becoming emotionally involved.[1]

Work at it for several reasons. It is one way of admitting that you are a stutterer. It is also a way of finding out how people react to stuttering and will help you realize that they are usually kind and tolerant. And it will give you the satisfaction of knowing that you have the courage to tackle your problem in an obvious way.[2]

It is also helpful if you inject a little humor or even are willing to joke about your stuttering.[3]

Doing this also helps reduce sensitivity. For instance, occasionally you might advertise the fact that you are a stutterer or make some joking remark about your stuttering[4]—such as explaining that if you didn't talk you wouldn't stutter—or announce "there may be a brief intermission due to technical difficulties." These remarks aren't very funny, are they? Probably not to you as a stutterer, but they may be to others.

It is helpful to develop a sense of humor about your difficulty.[5] At the same time, do not go overboard and laughingly and fraudently pretend that your stuttering is funny, as some stutterers have done, while feeling terrible about it inside.

---

[1]Now I am going to ask you to do a strange thing: *to stutter on purpose.* I know it sounds weird but it works. Why? Because it helps drain away the fear (what have you got to hide if you are willing to stutter on purpose?) and it provides a lot of experience practicing the act of stuttering in a highly voluntary and purposeful manner. The more you stutter on purpose, the less you hold back; and the less you hold back, the less you stutter. (Emerick)

[2]By gradually learning to stutter on purpose and without pain (the stutterer) will lose a lot of the negative emotions that color his disorder; when this occurs, he'll find great relief. (Van Riper)

[3]Consider humor as you look at your mistakes in speaking. Many things about stuttering can be funny. (Neely)

[4]One way to make your listener feel at ease about your stuttering is to tell an occasional joke about it. (Trotter)

[5]Make fun of your stuttering and yourself. The best of all humor is self-directed. (Emerick)

Your willingness to stutter, particularly in a modified way, is a very powerful aspect of therapy that can help lead to a most lasting and satisfying change in fluency.[1]

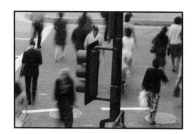

---

[1]The stutterer must be willing to be purposely abnormal. (Hulit)

Avoidance is the heart and core of stuttering. Avoidance behavior—holding back—is essential for the maintenance of stuttering behavior. Stuttering simply cannot survive a total weakening of avoidance, coupled with a concerted strengthening of approach tendencies. If there is no holding back there is no stuttering. (Sheehan)

Eliminating Secondary Symptoms

This fourth guideline suggests that you eliminate—that is stop doing—any secondary behaviors or unnecessary mannerisms which you may exhibit when stuttering or trying to avoid difficulty.[1] Possibly you have no such irregular behaviors, although most stutterers do.

This rule does not apply to the abnormal activity of your speech muscles or mechanism which is covered under rule (7). It refers to other noticeable, unnecessary or accessory body movements which may characterize the particular pattern of your stuttering.

They are what speech pathologists call secondary symptoms, and they refer to actions which are not necessary for the production of speech: physical mannerisms such as eye blinking, fixations, nostril or facial grimaces, mouth protrusions or postures, covering your mouth with your hand, head movements or scratching, jaw jerks, ear pulling, finger snapping or tapping, coin jingling, knee slapping, foot tapping or shuffling, hand movements, or what have you.[2]

Such irregular movements may have started because at one time they seemed to help you get through a block or enabled you to avoid trouble. But now they may have

---

[1] I feel that the stutterer's first task in speech correction is to learn to stop the physical struggle with which he has formerly met his speech blocks. (Bluemel)

[2] John's habitual pattern consisted of a violent tilting back of his head; rolling his eyes toward the ceiling; the muscles of his neck would stand out; he would become flushed; he would twist his face in a forced grimace; attempt various starters; some head jerks in an effort to release himself from the blocks and would also accompany his stuttering with various body gestures. (Sheehan)

become part of the stuttering itself. You will be happier when you eliminate any such unnecessary and unattractive actions.[1]

Of course you may not be guilty of doing such things, but you need to get rid of any such habits you do have. It is essential to learn to modify and control them. But before you can tackle them, of course, you need to find out what you do.[2]

This involves observing yourself when you stutter or when you are trying not to. These habits are usually automatic and involuntary, and you may not even realize when such symptoms are occurring.

It's not easy to scrutinize yourself and become fully aware of habits which you have been using to avoid difficulty and which you may have accumulated over the years. You cannot see yourself stuttering, but you should be able to feel what you do. Or you can ask a member of your family or a close friend to watch when you stutter and make notes after you have described what to look for.

You could start by picking out in advance some specific speaking situations which will occur today or tomorrow. Resolve to study yourself as carefully as possible on these occasions. Watch out for any unnecessary movements you make when stuttering or when expecting to. Disregard any normal gestures but make sure they are normal and not used to beat time with the speech attempt or to jerk out of your stutter.

---

[1] The job is to think and work in a positive manner. The job involves coming to realize that these head jerks, eye blinks, tongue clicks…are not helping to get those words out. They are preventing the words from being said strongly, aggressively and fluently. (Rainey)

[2] Make an inventory of speech related struggle that accompanies your stuttering. (Moses)

Here's where a mirror, particularly a full-length mirror, will come in handy to help you observe yourself. If you have difficulty talking on the phone, make some phone calls while watching yourself in the mirror.[1] Note any or all irregular movements (or postures) associated with your stuttering. Don't skip any of them. To double check make phone calls which will be particularly embarrassing and will put pressure on you. After each situation, make a list of symptoms in your workbook.[2]

You should have little trouble identifying and listing a conspicuous secondary symptom, but it may be a little more difficult to spot others. Stutterers can be unaware of behaviors which may be obvious to others. You may be surprised to find that you are doing something you would not do if you didn't stutter or expect to. So while you are working on this rule, make a point of observing yourself as carefully as possible.

Of course, if possible, it is even more advantageous in studying your secondary symptoms to have videotapes made of the way you talk. This enables you to both see and hear yourself at the same time.

(This guideline does not suggest that a stutterer should stop using any normal gestures which he has been in the habit of using to add expression or emphasis to his conversation. In fact, normal gesturing is encouraged as long as it is not timed to a beat or timing of one's speech.)

Getting rid of any secondary symptoms you may have should be a definite goal. In doing so, you will be getting rid of crutches which may have originally helped you get the word out but which can give no permanent relief.

---

[1] For example, you can look at yourself in the mirror and assess what you are doing while you make a phone call likely to elicit stuttering. (Murray)

[2] Begin by listing the struggle behaviors that you use which are not part of the act of speaking. You will seek to eliminate these behaviors by increasing your awareness of them and separating them from your attempts to talk. (Moses)

How to Work on Secondary Symptoms

How do you go about eliminating such behavior? It may not be easy. Sometimes such a habit can be so compulsive that it's almost impossible to stop.[1] But you can stop it if you make up your mind to do so. You can't stop stuttering by will power, but if you are determined, you can get rid of secondary symptoms by disciplining yourself to do so. But one needs to go about it in a systematic manner.

Unfortunately, there are no universal secondary symptoms which are common to all stutterers. You might blink your eyes, swing your arms, protrude your lips, jingle your coins, blow your nose, or make some kind of timing movement, etc. It could be anything. Also the problems of others may be different from yours, but that is not important since they will just be used as examples and the principles of correction outlined should apply to all such stuttering habits or tricks.

> Crutches...can give no permament relief.

Anyway, let's start by selecting some movement you make which you would like to correct. Even if there is more than one, it is better to work on only one at a time.

One way to start bringing it under control is to consciously make such movements **purposely** while not talking. For instance, if you have the habit of swinging your arm in trying to talk, then it is suggested that you practice swinging your arm intentionally while alone and not talk-

---

[1] Get rid of these artificial devices! This may seem impossible at first, but depend on your own natural resources and you will find that in the final analysis you will be greatly rewarded. (Barbara)

ing. And then start talking to yourself and swinging your arm but varying its speed and action so you can feel yourself consciously doing it in a different way.[1]

Or, for instance, if you have the habit of blinking your eyes, do it purposely in your accustomed manner when alone and not talking. And then, when talking to yourself, consciously and purposely vary the timing or speed of the blink. This approach to such problems calls for you to do these things purposely in a concentrated manner. Bringing such a habit under conscious control will make it easier to manage or restrain.

Practice taking control of these habits in anxiety-producing situations until you know you are the master and can skip it altogether. The basic idea is to make the behavior voluntary while it is occurring—then to vary it voluntarily—then to curtail its duration—then to stutter on the word without it. You can stop these mannerisms if you are determined to do so.

As an example, you might be interested in how one stutterer eliminated a rather grotesque secondary symptom of head jerking. This is how he did it.

"I'd always hated my head jerking. Looked awful, I know, and it bothered other people but I'd never been able to control it until now. It just seemed to take off when I blocked hard. I suffered from it for many years but it's gone now. I've learned how to keep it out and now my fear of stuttering has gone way down and I'm not stuttering much.

"Here's how I did it. It was suggested that I watch myself in the mirror when making phone calls. At first I could not bear to look at my jerking in the mirror but kept at it and

---

[1]Set up a program of change. Take all the different elements that make up your stuttering pattern, e.g. head jerks, eye blinks, etc. Then consciously and deliberately attempt to add (exaggerate), vary (instead of jerking your head to the right, jerk it to the left) and drop out the separate parts one at a time. Break up the stereotyped nature of how you go about doing your stuttering. (Emerick)

finally got curious about it. So I studied it. I found that I jerked it suddenly and always to the right side. It occurred only after I tensed my jaw and neck greatly and only after a series of fast repetitions. Why did I always have to let it jerk to the right? What happened just before the jerk? I noticed that I also squinted one eye (the right one) just before it happened. I found that on my easier blockings my eye didn't squint.

"Well, then I began to change these things. I made more phone calls and tried to jerk my head in the same way but on words I wasn't afraid of, and more slowly and on purpose. Then when the real head-jerking occurred, I tried jerking it to the **left** or moving my head and jaw slowly rather than swiftly. I found I could change and control it and when I did, I didn't feel helpless. I got so I could change the involuntary jerk into a voluntary one.

"Then I was no longer a slave to the habit but the master. Also by slowing down the repetitions that preceded it, I discovered that I could prevent it from happening. There was one other thing that I did too that helped greatly. I experimented with relaxing my jaw and neck when beginning to stutter. Couldn't always do it, but when I did I found I could keep my head steady and in control. What a relief! I've got a long way to go but at least when I stutter I'm no longer that abnormal monster I once was."

Another stutterer had a habit of tapping his foot when he stuttered, sort of beating time to the word or syllable.[1] To find out how bad it was and exactly what he was doing, he picked out some speaking situations and counted the number

---

[1]To me syllable-tapping was an old story that had no happy ending. I had tried it in junior high and high school, using an ordinary lead pencil. Vividly I recall my embarrassment when I pressed too hard and the pencil lead flew high in the air, to everyone's amusement but mine. After that I tapped for awhile on the eraser end, then gave it up completely, so I thought. But finger-tapping remained a part of my instrumental stuttering pattern for many ensuing years. (Sheehan)

of times he tapped his foot when stuttering. It was most difficult for him to do this, but he finally was able to get a count and discovered that they usually came on certain words or sounds when he was under stress.

Then he experimented with over-tapping more than he ordinarily would. He also practiced tapping purposely when he did not stutter, although he had to be particularly careful to be sure it was done voluntarily. The idea, of course, was to bring his compulsive tapping under conscious control. Then he worked on varying the way he tapped when he was stuttering by doing it differently than he ordinarily would. He would plan ahead of time how he would vary it so that he could have the feeling of its being under his control.

Do you get the idea? In order to work on eliminating a secondary symptom it is important to investigate it down to the smallest detail. You need to understand what you are doing before you can expect to win the battle against any such habit.[1] As you gain this knowledge, then start to vary your behavior. It is always helpful to purposely act out your symptom (whatever it may be) when you are not stuttering.

The key to eliminating it is to get it under conscious control from an involuntary movement to a voluntary movement. If you forget and find that you are not in control, then start over again. As you talk, voluntarily vary the way you do it on purpose. Practice taking over control in anxiety producing situations until you know you are the master and can skip it altogether.

The basic idea is to make the behavior voluntary while it is occurring—then to vary it voluntarily—then to shorten its duration—then to stutter on the word without it. You can stop these mannerisms if you are determined to do so.

---

[1] The mannerism should be closely observed in the mirror, studied, analyzed, imitated, practiced and deliberately modified. (Johnson)

Pay enough attention to the things you do that interfere with your normal speech, the things that you do that you call your stuttering, to understand that they are unnecessary and to change or eliminate them. (Johnson)

Rule (5)   *(page 46)*

Eliminating Avoidances, Postponements and Substitutions

This particularly important guideline calls for you to make a real effort to eliminate—that means stop—any and all avoidance, substitution or postponement habits which you may have acquired to put off, hide or minimize your stuttering. It is very important for you to develop speech that is avoidance-free.

This may present more of a problem than you think since much of a stutterer's abnormal behavior may be traced to his efforts to postpone or avoid what he considers threatening situations.[1,2] Many stutterers feel they must be ready for every eventuality so they can avoid the danger of getting stuck.[3]

While temporarily affording relief, avoidances will actually increase your fears and cause you more trouble in the long run.[4] They keep it aroused until time runs out or their effectiveness wears out. Stuttering will be perpetuated by successful avoidances.

---

[1]Your pattern of stuttering behavior consists chiefly of the things you are doing to avoid stuttering. (J. D. Williams)

[2]What you call your stuttering consists mostly of the tricks, the crutches you use to cover up. (Sheehan)

[3]The stutterer believes that the most important communication in speech is to avoid stuttering at all costs. (Trotter)

[4]What happens is this: The successful avoidance causes some anxiety reduction. Then, when a similar situation presents itself, the need to avoid is even stronger due to the preceding reinforcement. But now, no avoidance is possible. The conflict becomes even greater. And so several vicious circles (or rather spirals) are set into motion. (Van Riper)

Why shouldn't you avoid saying your name, or avoid answering the phone when you feel that you might stutter doing so? Or why isn't it all right to at least temporarily postpone doing something? Or why shouldn't you substitute a more easily said word for one on which you might stutter? Why not?

There is one good reason for not doing these things—and it is a powerful one. The more you make a practice of avoiding, postponing or substituting, the more you will keep on using such crutches to avoid trouble; and they will just reinforce your fear of stuttering. Why keep building up fear? If there is one thing the stutterer needs more than anything else, it is to reduce his fears and certainly not to reinforce them. Avoidance only makes the fear of stuttering worse.[1,2]

There are many different avoidance tactics to which stutterers sometimes resort in their attempts to minimize or escape trouble such as dodging speaking situations, avoiding social contacts or talking on the phone, using secondary symptoms or exaggerated gestures, talking more rapidly, repeating words or going back to get a running start, talking in a monotone or sing-song voice, varying the pitch or intensity of the voice, affecting unnaturally aggressive behavior, acting like a clown, writing down what needs to be said, playing dumb or hard-of-hearing, etc.

Avoidances reinforce your fear of stuttering.

---

[1]Avoidance only increases fear and stuttering and must be reduced. (Czuchna)

[2]And what actually happens is that the more you cover-up and try to avoid stuttering the more you will stutter. (Barbara)

Postponements include various stalling devices such as clearing the throat, swallowing, coughing, blowing the nose, putting in unnecessary words such as 'you know' or 'I mean,' or 'that is,' or making excessive use of interjections like 'uh,' 'er,' 'well,' waiting for someone to supply the word, etc. Substitutions involve using synonyms, easy words or other phrases for those on which you think you might block.[1] Or you may sneak up on a feared word from a different direction or adopt other strategies. Postponements and substitutions are variations of avoidance practices.

As has been pointed out, stuttering is what the stutterer does in trying not to stutter. So, if you could willingly and wholeheartedly adopt an attitude of not trying to cover up or avoid, it would make a world of difference in the amount of trouble you have.[2,3]

This step will require concentrated effort and may not be easy. It is suggested that you read, study and put to work assignments such as those listed in this next section.

How to Work on Avoidances

Conforming to this rule and eliminating all your avoidance practices may be a tough assignment, but many authorities feel that a non-avoidance attitude will give you more relief than any other therapy procedure. So let's make

---

[1] In shunning difficult words the stammerer has recourse to synonyms, circumlocutions and evasions. With the adult stutterer the use of synonyms becomes a standard method of escaping the speech impediment. One stammerer says facetiously that he has learned the whole dictionary in order to have synonyms available. (Bluemel)

[2] Working on my own I set about to eliminate every last vestige of avoidance of words and situations. (Sheehan)

[3] Be determined to reduce your use of avoidances. (Moses)

an all-out effort to stop any and all avoidance habits or tricks you may have acquired to put off, hide or minimize your stuttering.[1,2]

Your first step should be to work on finding out to what extent, when and how you may be using avoidances, so you will know what needs to be changed. Plan to start in the morning to observe yourself carefully as you go through the day in order to discover and identify what avoidance tricks you may be using.

Study your thought and action during the day, and make notes in your workbook of what you did and why you did it. Take note of what actions or lack of action were influenced by your concern about avoiding trouble. Compile this information for several days. You will be surprised at the number of times you avoid, postpone or substitute.

After compiling this information, you should start to work on trying to correct all such practices. It may be too difficult to attempt to work on all of them at the same time, so a gradual approach may be better although that's a matter for your own judgment.

Anyway, pick out one avoidance habit which you know is undesirable and decide to go to work on it. Make a real effort to counteract that particular habit only. Go about it in as systematic a way as possible. You will need to watch yourself for some time to make sure that it gets adequate

---

[1]The habitual avoidance of speaking situations and feared words will get you nowhere in the long run. (Murray)

[2]Like many of you, one of the most common and debilitating characteristics of my problem was the habit of avoiding.... There was almost no limit to what I would do to avoid situations in which I feared my stuttering would embarrass me. Going to a party would be an extremely tiring event because the entire evening would be spent trying to stay alert for words on which I might stutter and finding ways to avoid them. (Luper)

attention so that you won't use it any more. Make notes of your accomplishments as well as your failures.[1] Such changes don't just happen, so don't let yourself become discouraged by the difficulties encountered. Persevere at the task.

For instance, resolve that you will not substitute words.[2,3] To do this, you will have to watch yourself carefully because you may be doing it frequently. One way to approach a substitution problem is to deliberately use words on which you would expect to stutter. Say what you have to say, and if you stutter, still persevere. Write out the exact words you are about to say. And say them without substitution or revision.

Or for instance, there is no advantage in pretending not to hear when someone speaks to you—nor should you stand mute pretending to think of an answer—nor say that you do not know when you do know.[4] Nor should you dodge speaking situations—or avoid social responsibilities—or give up speech attempts or leave the scene of approaching trouble.[5]

---

[1]Make a list of all your avoidances. What types do you use (starters, delaying tactics, etc.)? When, and in what context do you use them? How frequently do you resort to evasion? In other words, prepare an avoidance inventory. Then, systematically vary and exaggerate each one; use the avoidances when you don't need to in a highly voluntary manner. Finally, when you find yourself using an avoidance involuntarily, invoke a self-penalty; for example, if you avoid the word "chocolate," you must then use that word several times immediately thereafter. One of the best penalties is to explain to the listener the avoidance you have just used and why you should resist such evasions. (Emerick)

[2]The author knows from his own past experience as a severe stutterer and from his dealings with many other stutterers, that it is better to have a five-minute blocking than to avoid a word successfully. We never conquer fear by running away; we only increase it. (Van Riper)

[3]The thing that discouraged me most was the realization that I could no longer detour around a difficult bugaboo word with the substitution of a clever synonym. (Wedberg)

[4]You sometimes create the impression of aloofness, unfriendliness, or stupidity when you are in reality friendly and well-informed. (Johnson)

[5]At times you may totally avoid stuttering by choosing to be absent, by withdrawing from a speaking situation, or while speaking you may substitute a non-feared word (one on which you do not expect to stutter) for a feared one. This allows you to escape for the moment, but increases the worry about future situations. (J. D. Williams)

One approach would be for you to make a point of talking more in feared situations. Possibly search out one feared situation every day and go into it, being sure to watch out that you do not back down and dodge the situation after you have determined to follow through. Then write out a description of the experience.

This does not mean that you need to volunteer to make speeches before an audience, but you will feel better about yourself when you deliberately enter more speaking situations.[1] For example, ask the bus driver how much the fare is even if you know. Or say "good morning" to a store clerk when you previously said nothing.

As you progress, you will be encouraged to participate in situations that offer a challenge. You need to talk as much as possible.[2,3] Sooner or later you will have to stop running away. Now is a good time to stand and fight.

Actually, you will feel a sense of achievement by voluntarily seeking out feared words and entering difficult situations. The less you avoid, the more confidence you will have in yourself as a respectable and worthy person. In the give and take of normal life, you should not back down but speak up.[4,5]

---

[1] Enter more speaking situations. (D. Williams)

[2] One way of reducing your fear is by increasing the amount of speaking you do, particularly in situations that you customarily avoid. (Trotter)

[3] Search for those words and situations that are beginning to bug you rather than hiding them until they build up giant fears. (Luper)

[4] The habitual avoidance of speaking situations and feared words will get you nowhere in the long run. (Murray)

[5] Don't let yourself avoid speaking because you might stutter. (Guitar)

Using the Telephone

Did the phone just ring? Don't push others away so you can answer it, but if you would normally be the logical person to take the call, do so. This may be tackling your biggest fear.[1] Perhaps you say to yourself that it's too much, and you just can't do it. Even if you are not trying to overcome your stuttering, you can not expect to go through life always avoiding the telephone. Sooner or later, you'll have to pick up that receiver and talk. The longer you put it off, the harder it will be.[2]

On the other hand, perhaps it doesn't bother you to talk on the phone, but you have other problems. Let's assume that you did answer that call just now and you talked to the person at the other end of the line. During the conversation, did you come to a word on which you expected to stutter and then did you think of another way of saying it to avoid trouble on that word? Possibly you did. If so, you added another brick to the wall of your fear.

Incidentally, when you saw so-and-so the other day and you were afraid you might stutter talking to him, what did you do? How did you get around speaking to him? Did you cross to the other side of the room or did you hide from him—or did you just clam up? Unfortunately, we do not know what sort of contacts or meetings you avoid.

As we said before, when you run into normal situations when you would like to talk, make a point of taking advantage of them and speak up.[3,4] Your opinions need to be heard

---

[1] I remember well how often I "played-deaf" when the telephone would ring. Sometimes, unfortunately, I might be standing not more than a few feet from the ringing telephone and my protestations regarding "answer the telephone" would be of no avail. (Adler)

[2] Guidelines for using the telephone on page 147.

[3] One of the things we were forced to do to reduce our avoidances was to make ourselves talk more, especially in feared situations. (Murray)

[4] One way of reducing your fear is by increasing the amount of speaking you do, particularly in situations that you customarily avoid. (Trotter)

as well as those of the next person. Use whatever words come to you. Plan to express your thoughts without making substitutions or revisions to avoid stuttering.[1] If you have the determination to tackle your problems in this way, you will build confidence in yourself.

As you have had the habit of planning how to avoid trouble, now spend time planning how not to avoid trouble. At times you may fail to follow through but if you do, you should make up for such failures by entering other or similar situations in which you are afraid you might stutter.[2] No one wins all the time but one can always recoup. In any case, be honest with yourself regarding any such assignments.[3] If you alibi, you are kidding no one but yourself.

Here's an account of what one stutterer did in trying to reduce the avoidances that constantly reinforced his fears, as he tells it.

"For years I've been using every imaginable trick I could think of to keep from stuttering or to hide it when it came. Most of the time I can get away with it, but even so I live with the fear that sooner or later I will be unmasked and I usually am. But the worst of it is the constant vigilance I've got to keep, the constant sizing up of situations and sentences for signs of approaching trouble. I get so tired of always having to get ready to duck and dodge and cover up this constant fear.

---

[1] Search for those words and situations that are beginning to bug you rather than hiding them until they build up giant fears. (Luper)

[2] Deliberately enter previously feared situations. (Moses)

[3] We never conquer fear by running away from it; we only increase it. (Van Riper)

"Anyway today, thoroughly fed up, I decided to attack the situation head-on. I began by going to a cafe for breakfast rather than the cafeteria where I've always gone so I wouldn't have to talk. I walked past the cafe three times before getting up enough courage to walk in, but I finally did.

"I found myself rehearsing my order, changing my selections so I might not stutter, but I was so disgusted with my weakness that when the waitress came I just blurted out 'b-b-b-bacon and eggs!' and stuttered on purpose on bacon. I looked at her and she didn't bat an eye. Just asked me if I wanted coffee and I said again 'b-b-b-bacon and eggs and coffee.' I can't tell you how good I felt. For once I hadn't been a coward. If they don't like it, they can lump it! I felt strong, not weak and I sure enjoyed the bacon and eggs.

"After breakfast I was feeling so good about myself that I decided to tackle the phone which has always been my most feared situation. I wanted to find out when the buses left for Trenton, and ordinarily I might have gone to the bus station rather than phone. That phone fear is terrible, and I hung up twice when they answered before saying a word. I was in such a panic I hardly knew what I wanted to say even if I could have started.

"So I sat down and wrote out the words 'When do the buses leave for Trenton this afternoon?,' put the mirror by the phone so I could see myself, dialed the number and then said it word by word. I stuttered though not as much as I'd expected, and I had to say it twice because the clerk didn't understand the first time but I got the information I needed. Felt all drained out afterwards but also triumphant. I'll lick this thing yet."

So can you.[1]

---

[1]Keep in mind that...the less you avoid words and situations, the less you will stutter in the long run. (J. D. Williams)

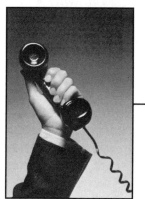

Keep in mind that…the less you
avoid words and
situations, the less
you will stutter in the
long run.

(J. D. Williams)

Rule (6) *(page 48)*

Maintaining Eye Contact

If you are like many stutterers, you probably do not look people squarely in the eye when you talk to them. Chances are that if you observe yourself carefully, you will find that you usually avert your eyes, particularly when you are stuttering or anticipating a block. And by doing so, you tend to increase any feelings of shame or embarrassment you may have about your difficulty.

Maintaining eye contact will not of itself stop your stuttering, but it will help reduce feelings of shyness and tend to build self-confidence. It is this sensitivity which generates much of the tension which causes or aggravates your trouble. So this guideline calls for you to establish the habit of eye contact with your listener.[1,2]

This doesn't mean that you need to stare fixedly at the person to whom you are talking, but still you should look the other person squarely in the eye more or less continuously. Establish eye contact before you begin to speak and continue to do so in a natural way. Particularly, do your best not to look away when you stutter or expect to.

It is possible that you already practice good eye contact, but more probably you are embarrassed and do not. Remember, it is difficult to observe yourself so do your best to be honest with yourself. You might ask someone with whom you converse, such as a member of your family, to watch and find out if you shift your eyes just before or when you stutter.

---

[1]You must acquire the ability to keep good eye contact with your listener throughout your moment of stuttering. (Van Riper)

[2]Develop eye control with your audience and create a friendly atmosphere. (Barbara)

Perhaps you look away because you are afraid that your listener will react with pity, rejection or impatience. This is not apt to be true. Using eye contact will enable you to test the validity of your fears, and it should put your listener more at ease. Moreover, by maintaining eye contact you can demonstrate that you are accepting—not rejecting—your stuttering as a problem to be solved.[1] When you look away, you are denying the problem.

Look the world squarely in the eye.

Anyway, do your best to maintain good eye contact as a habit. You will feel better for doing so, as it will help you combat feelings of inferiority and self-consciousness. Therapists recommend its use in trying to help people who are shy and bashful. Interpersonal communication is always facilitated by eye contact, even if you don't stutter.[2] Good speakers use it naturally.

It is unnecessary to turn or hang your head in shame which may be what you are doing unconsciously when you avert your eyes. We hope you can develop a feeling of self-confidence that you are as good as the next person. Do your best to look the world squarely in the eye.

How to Go About Maintaining Eye Contact

Following through on this rule may represent more of a problem than you think. Many stutterers have become so shy that it is difficult for them to look anybody straight in the eye when they are stuttering. It is suggested that you

---

[1]The value of eye contact is the effect it has on the stutterer. It almost forces him to keep the stuttering going forward through the word. It's an assertive behavior and a positive act. It's hard to withdraw and back off if you are holding eye contact. (Starbuck)

[2]Try to maintain eye contact with your listeners. Looking away severs the communication link with your audience and convinces them that you are ashamed and disgusted with the way you talk. (Moses)

double-check yourself carefully as you try the following procedures.

Start by looking at yourself in the mirror when alone and faking an easy block. Do you keep eye contact with yourself or do you avert your eyes? Try this repeatedly, making sure that you don't look away. Then do it when making a severe block. If you find you do not keep eye contact before and during the block, work at it until you find that you can and continue doiong it.

Then make some phone calls looking at yourself in the mirror while you are having real blocks. Watch yourself until you can talk without shifting your eyes during five or more real stutterings.[1] To complete this program successfully, this is a necessary step.

As you become more sure of yourself, it will be easier for you to maintain eye contact while talking in general conversation.[2] This does not mean that you have to stare fixedly or glare at your listeners, but look at them in a normal, natural way, and though they look away, continue to keep contact.

While talking to others, collect one, two, and then three occasions in which you maintain good eye contact as you are stuttering. Then make it ten occasions.

To prove that you have followed through, it is suggested you write down the names and eye colors of ten people with whom you have stuttered, or write down ten or more words on which you stuttered without losing normal, natural eye contact.

---

[1] Read a sentence, look up into the mirror, paraphrase the sentence while maintaining eye contact. (Adler)

[2] Be sure you don't look down or away at the moment of stuttering. Some people will look away no matter how much you try to keep contact. To succeed it is sufficient that you look at them. (Sheehan)

Use your ingenuity in devising other pertinent assignments. Build confidence in your ability to speak with good natural eye contact on all occasions from now on, and you will feel better for doing so. It will give you satisfaction to know that you can comply with this rule and will make you a more effective conversationalist.

Rule (7)   *(page 49)*

Finding Out What You Do
When You Stutter

An important part of this therapy program involves your finding out exactly what you are doing with your speech mechanism when you are having difficulty.[1] So you are asked to identify and feel the articulatory movements and the contacts which you do incorrectly when you are stuttering.[2]

The more you study how you block on certain sounds or words, the more you will realize that you can find ways to move through them without struggling. In other words, the more you carefully analyze your faulty speech habits, the more you should be able to take advantage of controls which will modify or eliminate your unnatural or unnecessary actions.[3,4]

Maybe you hate to even think about examining the way you stutter, but this information is important. Probably you have only a vague idea of how you stutter and can not duplicate your abnormalities.[5] Possibly all you know is that sometimes you speak freely, and at other times you get miserably stuck.

---

[1]Perhaps the first concrete step you should take is to acquaint yourself with your stuttering behavior. (Murray)

[2]How you stutter is terribly important. (Sheehan)

[3]The better your understanding of your speech problem and of what you yourself are doing that complicates the problem, the more you can do to help yourself feel capable of dealing with it successfully. (Johnson)

[4]It is important that you learn as much as possible about how you stutter and what you do when you stutter so that you can modify the symptoms. (Boland)

[5]Early in my therapy program, I made a startling discovery. Although I had stuttered for years, I really did not know much about what I did with my speech apparatus as I stuttered. (Luper)

In any case, we want you to get the feel of the actions of the muscles controlling your breath, mouth, lips and tongue so you can learn how to duplicate your stuttering and make a comparison with their action when you speak without trouble.[1]

Assignments will include studying speech muscle articulation and actions used in the formation of speech sounds and words when stuttering, as compared with their specific activity when you speak without difficulty.

To find this out, you will be asked to stutter on purpose, imitating your usual pattern and observing yourself in the mirror while doing it. And if, by any chance you have been able to have recordings or videotapes made of your stuttering, they will be of real help. To be able to both hear and see yourself stuttering will make it easier for you to study how to change or correct what you have been doing wrong.

Such assignments may seem strange and unpleasant, but progress is possible if you face up to and confront your problem, no matter how distressing it may be.[2,3] Others see and hear you stutter and if they can bear with it, so can you. It's not as bad as you imagine it.

---

[1]It is helpful for the stutterer to learn to analyze and identify the specific movements or lack of movements involved in his stuttering behavior. He will learn this by attending carefully to his behavior, e.g. what he is doing with his tongue, jaw and lips as he is stuttering. Then he can have a basis for comparison between what he needs to do to talk and what he is doing to interfere with that process. Most importantly, he can learn that he is doing things to interfere with talking, and hence he can learn to change them. (D. Williams)

[2]Another most important goal in your search for an ultimate cure is to acquaint yourself with your stuttering behavior. (Barbara)

[3]It is difficult to achieve a lasting change in stuttering if stutterers cannot quickly and correctly identify when they are stuttering. Unless they can do this, we think it is difficult to lastingly change stuttering. (Conture)

Analyzing the Pattern of Your Blocks

You are urged to conduct a self-examination and investigate your blocks so you can develop a feeling or sense of awareness of the movement and positions of your speech mechanism when you are stuttering.[1,2,3,4] This applies particularly to the things that you do which are unnatural and unnecessary.

How do you conduct this self-examination? One way to get a feeling of what is happening is to stutter extremely slowly when you block. This does not refer to talking slowly—but **stuttering slowly.**

When you anticipate trouble, go ahead and stutter, but do it in such slow motion that you have time to get the feel of exactly what you are doing wrong with your speech muscles.

Keep doing this, trying to sense what happens when you block and when making the transition to the next sound until you become aware of what is happening on those sounds which give you trouble. Make note, and record those things which you find are different and unnecessary.[5]

---

[1]Look and listen closely and discover just what it is that you are doing when you stutter. (Rainey)

[2]You've got to examine and analyze the act of speaking to see what errors you're making. What are you doing wrong that makes your speech come out as stuttering? (Starbuck)

[3]Perhaps the first concrete step you should take is to acquaint yourself with your stuttering behavior…. In order to carry this out effectively, you must first learn to keep in touch with yourself during your moments of stuttering…. Feedback of various types will assist you in this self-study endeavor. (Murray)

[4]When a moment of stuttering occurs it can be studied and its evil effects erased as much as possible. (Conture)

[5]As honestly as you can, try to observe yourself and write down your observations. (J. D. Williams)

Another way to get this information is to repeat your blocks when you have trouble. Be courageous and stutter on them over again. But the second time go through the block in such slow motion that you can get the feel of how your speech muscles are acting up.

Using a Mirror to Check Your Stutter

If you have trouble talking on the telephone, the use of a mirror offers you an excellent opportunity of observing what you are doing wrong when you stutter.[1,2] Place the mirror near the phone, located so that you can watch your face closely.

Then, of course, make some phone calls. If you have no one to contact, you can always call stores or offices asking for information while you monitor your stuttering. Then as you talk, watch the movements of your mouth, etc., and identify specifically the irregular or unnatural movements you make with your speech muscles.

Here again, if you can make a point of stuttering slowly, it will give you a better chance to see what is taking place. Also, if you can, freeze your action as you block, as it would help to make any unnatural positions more obvious.[3] You need this information so that you can imitate any unusual movements.

---

[1]For example you can look at yourself in a mirror and assess what you are doing while you make a phone call likely to elicit stuttering. (Murray)

[2]Watching yourself stutter in a mirror makes you more objective and less emotional about your stuttering. (Trotter)

[3]A simple way to apply this principle in the treatment of stuttering is to have the stutterer maintain or prolong or continue any given position of the speech mechanism that may occur at any stage of what he terms stuttering. (Johnson)

When off the phone, pick out a word that gives you trouble.[1] For example, it might be your name. Anyway, such a word will have a sound in it on which you frequently block.

As you observe yourself in the mirror, stutter purposely on the word, imitating the way you get stuck, making the block as realistic as possible.[2] Then repeat the block, stuttering on the sound or syllable only, but this time in extremely slow motion. It may be difficult to slow the stuttering down but keep working at it until you can do it slowly.

Now in order to make the comparison, utter the same sound again but correctly, trying to feel what happens when you produce the sound without stuttering as you look in the mirror. Say the syllable in slow motion many times until you become aware of the difference between the feel of your speech muscle activity when you block on it and when you say it fluently.[3] Make notes of the things you do that are different, not normal, or unnecessary when you stutter.

This may appear complex, but it should not be too difficult since you will probably find out that the way you stutter doesn't vary very much. You may find that your pattern of stuttering is more or less uniform and consistent, as most stutterers tend to repeat the same abnormal postures or speech muscle movements each time they stutter.

---

[1]Choose some words that begin with sounds that you think of as being hard—those on which you often stutter. (Aten)

[2]It turns out that a practical way for the stutterer to observe his own stuttering behavior is simply to duplicate it on purpose, imitate it, perform it, while watching himself in the mirror. (Johnson)

[3]To study your speech, analyze how you say words both fluently and in a stuttered form. (Neely)

Using a Tape Recorder to Help Check

A tape recorder can be of service in studying the way you stutter so that you can imitate it.[1] The recorder can be a small one, and inconspicuous, and its use need not be embarrassing—but even if it is evident, people are generally interested in observing how it works.[2]

Possibly you have already made recordings of conversations when talking with friends and members of your family. It is also desirable for you to take the recorder out and carry it around to make other recordings. If you do not want to talk with people you know, then make occasions to start conversations with strangers, even if only to ask the time of day or directions while you make recordings.[3]

As previously suggested, if you have trouble talking on the phone, you should make recordings of phone conversations in front of the mirror, sometimes freezing your articulations or continuing your repetitions, etc.[4] Then, of course, after you have recorded conversations, play the tapes back and listen to them.[5] Run the tapes slowly in those spots where you had trouble so you can have a better understanding of what happened.

---

[1] Listen to recordings of your speech. (Agnello)

[2] I would recommend the almost constant use of a tape recorder. There's nothing like being able to hear your own speech in order to judge what you do and don't like about it, and to decide what changes to make as you practice. Try to record your speech in different situations. (J. D. Williams)

[3] Another classic situation most stutterers fear is asking questions of strangers.... What I did, and have my patients do, is to stop people who are walking somewhere, or are in stores, and ask them questions concerning the time, directions, the price of some object, etc. (Adler)

[4] Listen to your own recording of this on tape and watch your performance of it in the mirror.... By listening to yourself stutter you accustom yourself to the sound of your stuttering. When you are in a real speaking situation and you hear yourself stutter, you're not as likely to panic. (Trotter)

[5] It is possible to record your speech in a communicative stressful situation, then play the tape back for the purpose of careful analysis. Painful as this may seem, it is a good way to bring yourself to grips with your problem. (Murray)

As you repeatedly do this, mimic (silently) or pantomime the actions of your speech muscles along with the recording. You need to see and hear and be able to duplicate what you are doing when you stutter. Work at this as best you can even if you have no recorder so you can have a much better understanding of the situation.[1]

Of course, it is even more advantageous if you can arrange to have videotapes made of your actions when you are stuttering. Viewing such tapes enables you to both see and hear what you are doing wrong which needs to be corrected. It puts you in the best position to study your difficulty. Obtaining such videotaping is recommended.

When you have discovered what you are letting your speech muscles do abnormally when you stutter, you can compare their activity with what they do when you speak fluently.[2] Completing this step may take a substantial amount of time, but keep at it until you feel you understand what you do incorrectly when you stutter.

Working to acquire the desired information of this step takes careful analysis, but the more insight you have about your difficulty, the easier it will be to solve it.[3] To give you more explicit examples of how you can check your speech muscle activities, read the next section describing how to analyze in detail what a stutterer does with his speech mechanism when he has difficulty. This section gives specific directions on how to study the errors you make. This information will show you how to make block corrections as described in the following chapters.

---

[1]In short, you need to develop a sharp sense of contrast between what you are doing that you call stuttering and what you do as you just talk easily. Use a mirror or a tape recorder to help you observe what you are doing. (D. Williams)

[2]You, as a stutterer, must study your speech patterns in order to become aware of the difference between stuttered and fluent speech. (Neely)

[3]When a moment of stuttering occurs it can be studied and its evil effects erased as much as possible. (Czuchna)

I am a stutterer. I am not like other people. I must think differently, act differently, live differently—because I stutter. Like other stutterers, like other exiles, I have known all my life a great sorrow and a great hope together, and they have made me the kind of person I am. An awkward tongue has molded my life.

(Johnson—written when he was a young man)

How to Analyze In Detail What You Do With Your Speech Mechanism When You Have Difficulty

This section describes in detail how you can feel and analyze your blocks to correct your errors.[1,2] Unfortunately, there is no way for us to know exactly what happens in your case. But we will list here some variations of stuttering behavior which may happen when certain consonant sounds are uttered. This will give you a better idea of how to study your problems.

It should first be noted that all vocal expression or speech is actually made up of separate and different sounds which are combined to make words.[3] To express it in another way, when you talk you articulate the sounds which form words. In the interest of simplicity, these sounds will be referred to as vowel and consonant sounds—the vowel sounds being 'a,' 'e,' 'i,' 'o,' 'u,' etc., and the consonant sounds 'b,' 'c,' 'd,' etc.

When you stutter, you may think that you are blocking on a word. That is true, but more specifically you are blocking on a sound of that word or in making the transition from one sound to the next in that word. To use a simple illustration when you stutter saying b-b-b-ball you are not just blocking on the "b" sound, as you have already sounded it, but having trouble making the **transition** to the rest of the word.

---

[1]You've got to examine and analyze the act of speaking to see what errors you are making. (Starbuck)

[2]At a time when you feel that you "are stuttering" pay very close attention to what you are doing.... You can ask yourself—precisely what are you doing? You should answer this question in descriptive detail, and when you have done this you should always ask yourself why you were doing what you were doing. (Johnson)

[3]You may think of a word as being a unit or lump of sound. Actually a word is composed of separate sounds much as a written word consists of separate letters. (Neely)

Many stutterers find their greatest difficulty in shifting from one sound to the next sound.

Among other possibilities, you may find out that your airflow is sporadic or jerky; or you let all your air out first and then try to talk without sufficient breath; or you use some kind of starter noises or interjections; or you jam your lips shut and can't get them apart; or your tongue sticks to the roof of your mouth; or you have rapidfire repetitions or just repeat sounds; or you have tremors in your jaw; or you have prolongation of certain sounds, etc.

Many find their greatest difficulty in shifting from one sound to the next...

Trying to Say a Name

Let's try out your speech muscle activity on a sample consonant sound. Let's assume that your name is Peter and you have particular trouble with the 'p' sound and the transition to the next sound.

(Virtually every stutterer has trouble with his own name, particularly when he is called on to identify himself to someone in authority.)

For your information the 'p' sound is called a "labial plosive." This kind of sound is correctly made by closing your lips and building up slight air pressure and then suddenly releasing the air by separating your lips quickly. Try making the sound by itself.

Anyway, now in front of your mirror, stutter badly on the 'p' sound as you say your name putting a lot of tension into it. Then stutter on it again in the same way but this time do it in extremely slow motion so you can have an opportunity to feel what your speech muscles are doing when you block. Repeat this several times.

What happened and what did you find out? Certainly you had an excessive amount of tension but where was it principally located? Perhaps there was no passage of air because your tight lips closed the airway.

Perhaps instead of attacking the 'p' sound directly, you hemmed and hawed, using various repetitive starter sounds like 'uh' or 'er' or 'well,' etc. Or maybe you stalled and started again repeating a phrase. Because of the tension, your speech muscles may have become temporarily frozen in a rigid position thus blocking any sound.

Possibly you had tiny vibrations in your lips or jaw—or possibly the sound came out p-p-p-p repetitively in a bounce pattern like a broken record. Or maybe your lips were squeezed or protruded and set in a fast vibration or trembling called tremor.

More likely you blocked because you held your mouth in a fixed position. In other words, you pressed your lips together so tightly on the 'p' sound that you couldn't separate them and let the air escape. You couldn't uncork your mouth because you were making such a hard, tight contact. Are you doing these things?

Of course you are not doing all these things and running into all these complications, but you need to write down how and where you get blocked making the 'p' sound as a reminder of what can be eliminated or modified.

Now, still in front of your mirror, say your name *without* stuttering in extremely slow motion repeatedly to get the feel of the difference between how you stutter on it and how you say it without stuttering. Feel the difference.

Anyway, let's make the assumption that your difficulty with the 'p' sound occurred because you pressed or squeezed your lips together so tightly or firmly that the sound was blocked. What can or should you do to change or correct that habit?

You can correct it by loosening or softening the tension in your lips in order to keep the pressure from building up. When you start to say your name relax your lips so they feel weak and flabby—and then consciously control your movement so that they come together only very slightly as you utter the 'p' sound.[1] This is called a light contact.

To produce a light contact, you have to control the action of your lip muscles so that they just barely touch with no pressure whatsoever. In this way, you can consciously control the action of your lips so that they touch only lightly as you allow the air from your breath to flow between them.[1] Practice making light, loose contacts so you can get the feel of maneuvering your lip movement through the 'p' sound.[2]

Using this as an example, your task is to figure out what kind of articulative contacts or movements you make when stuttering so you can learn how to change or control your speech muscle action.[3] This needs to be done to correct any of the bad habits you have acquired. You will find that many of them are fairly easy to understand and can be modified or eliminated through the application of corrective procedures described in the next chapters.[4]

---

[1]Concentrate on controlling the lip muscles so that they just barely touch and air is able to flow between them. (Starbuck)

[2]We must enable them to learn that it is possible to start a feared 'p' word, for example, without pressing the lips together with compulsive force. (Van Riper)

[3]As you say an isolated word beginning with a 'b' or 'p' for example, concentrate on the feeling of movement as you bring your lips together and as they move to the next sound. (Neely)

[4]You, too, can explore the unknown. When you do you may find that you push your lips too hard or jam your tongue against the roof of your mouth. (Luper)

Others are more complex; but if you analyze your faulty speech habits carefully, it is reasonable to expect that you should be able to use controls which will modify or eliminate your unnatural or unnecessary actions.[1]

The more you continue to study the way you stutter on the sounds and words on which you have difficulty and then compare them with how you say them fluently, the more you will realize that you should be able to move through a block easily without struggling.

Results from Comparison

From this comparison, you will find that you must have been making unnecessary speech movements that represent part of your difficulty. Such movements would not be needed for the correct production of the sounds or words you are trying to say. So now that you have studied and know what these needless or superfluous actions are, you are in a position to work on eliminating them.[2]

We wish we could specifically list what needs to be done in your case, but we are not familiar with the particular pattern of how you stutter. And unfortunately there are so many detail variations involved in the articulation of all sounds that it would be impossible to describe all of them.

Taking advantage of this information, the next chapters will explain how you can work on changing or correcting what is wrong by using block corrections. Even though it is impossible to consciously control all the speech actions

---

[1]The better your understanding of your speech problem, and of what you are doing to complicate the problem, the more you can do to help yourself feel capable of dealing with it successfully. (Johnson)

[2]The stutterer must be aware of articulatory postures and controls and varying degrees of muscular tension so that he can eliminate or modify behaviors which interfere with fluency. (Hulit)

involved, still by using these block corrections as described, you will find that you do not need to stutter as you have been doing.[1] We remind you again that stuttering is something you are doing, and you can vary or change what you are doing.

You can change your old stuttering response into a more appropriate one. There is no need for you to spend the rest of your life struggling with blocks and making yourself miserable. Have faith in your ability to conquer your problem.

---

[1]Once you begin to see what you are doing that makes talking difficult, you will find that much of this behavior is controllable. (Luper)

Block Corrections

As a result of your study in the last chapter, presumably you now more correctly understand precisely what you have been having your speech muscles do abnormally when you stutter. From your knowledge of this valuable information, of course, the next step is to take action to modify or correct what you have been doing unnecessarily or incorrectly. How is this done?

It is recommended that you now practice block corrections. There are three of these which are designed to show you how you can modify or change what you are doing as you stutter. And they will enable you to cope with your fluency disruptions and the fears associated with them.

The next three chapters describe how to work these corrections. The first one entitled "Post-Block Correction" explains in careful detail how you can correct what you have done abnormally **after** you have experienced a block.[1] This is most educational and should be practiced first.

The next chapter entitled "In-Block Correction" describes how best to pull out of a block which you may be experiencing. Then the chapter entitled "Pre-Block Correction" outlines how to prepare to move smoothly through a block which is anticipated.[2] That is the goal toward which your efforts have been directed and describes the final step in this program.

---

[1] By using the awareness of muscle movement to guide your lips, tongue and throat from sound to sound throughout the word. (Neely)

[2] The terms post-block correction, in-block correction and pre-block correction designate to the stutterer the proper time and sequence of applying procedures which lead to better speech. (Starbuck)

———————

...the behavior called stuttering is extremely modifiable. It is possible for the speaker to change drastically the things that he does that he calls his stuttering. (Johnson)

———————

Rule (8) *(page 51)*

Post-Block Correction

CANCELLATION

This is probably one of the best single procedures that you can use in learning how to stutter less severely. It is not complicated but it does make you confront and accept your stuttering.

Use this post-block correction procedure immediately after you have a block and before you continue with what you have to say. At that time it should be easier to feel exactly what went wrong, and how it should be modified.

Accordingly, it is recommended that you now put into effect the results of your findings of how you stutter by practicing these corrections, sometimes referred to as cancellations. Do your best to follow through on this. It offers an opportunity for immediately revising your behavior in order to correct your errors.[1]

Briefly, the post-block correction works as follows. After you stutter on a word, you are to pause momentarily to allow time for you to think back and figure out what you did which caused the stutter and plan how to correct it.[2] In making post-block corrections, you are called on to overcorrect your faulty speech muscle movements.

---

[1]You must learn how to cancel. This refers to a technique wherein you go right through your own stuttering block, then pause during which you study the block you have just had, then try the word in a different way. (Van Riper)

[2]In other words a post-block cancellation theoretically allows stutterers the opportunity to exercise and develop self-control where previously only lack of control prevailed. (Stromsta)

The following section outlines the sequence of action. Study the explanation carefully to be sure that you understand exactly how the process is executed, and then put it into effect when you stutter. The numbers in parentheses denote the steps in sequence.

Post-Block Correction—Sequence of Action

When you stutter on a word, the first thing you do is (1) finish saying the word on which you blocked—i.e., complete the entire word. Don't quit or use a trick to dodge it. Then (2) you have got to have the determination to pause—come to a complete stop once the word has been uttered. The pause is to give you time to study your problem and pantomime its solution.[1,2]

After you have stopped, (3) try to relax the tension in your speech mechanism, particularly in your throat. Get the feeling of your tongue lying limp in the bottom of your mouth. Let your jaw drop slightly open as if you were going to drool with your lips loose. The key is to feel the tension draining out as your breathing returns to normal.[3]

---

[1]The pause allows the stutterer to prepare his speech mechanism for modification by reducing muscular tension and by returning the articulation to a neutral position. (Hulit)

[2]As soon as the stutterer is able to be fairly consistent in pausing after his moment of stuttering, we ask him next to use the pause as an opportunity to try to calm himself and to begin the next word slowly. (Van Riper)

[3]Thinking of and striving for increased relaxation when under stress will provide a competing response which will help you be more calm. (Gregory)

As you pause and relax (4) think back and ask yourself what caused you to get stuck on that sound—what did you do wrong—what did you do that was abnormal.[1] In the past chapter you studied the mistakes you made when you blocked on different sounds and what you could do with your speech muscles to change or correct these errors. Using this information, think what went wrong when you stuttered and now (5) review what you can do to slowly reverse or change the errors you made on this particular sound or word.

Then (6) mentally rehearse or silently mimic how it would feel to have your mouth slowly make these corrections so as to modify your usual pattern of stuttering and move through the word.

(As you take time to study your blocking problem and plan how to deal with it, it may seem to you that the person to whom you are talking may lose interest in what you have to say. That is possible but stick to your guns, and concentrate on working this post-block correction properly. Take your time as the pause needs to be long enough to accomplish your purpose of preparing your course of action.[2])

---

[1]When the word is completed, stop completely and analyze all of the errors you made while all of the tensions and pressures are still fresh. (Starbuck)

[2]As stutterers begin to put these pauses into their speech following their moments of stuttering while appearing relatively unruffled and unhurried, they find much more acceptance from those with whom they are communicating than they had expected. (Van Riper)

After determining what you need to do to correct the errors you made—and after you have mentally rehearsed how it will feel to say the word again while making these corrections—then and only then—(7) repeat the word as you feel yourself making the corrections.

BUT, this time (8) articulate the sound on which you blocked in a smooth, prolonged manner. This will give you time to concentrate on feeling yourself correcting or at least changing the speech muscle errors you made when you stuttered. And keep your voice flowing to enable you to slowly make the transition to the next sound.[1]

In speaking this way please remember to over-correct your wrong speech muscle action. Change what you usually do when you block on a sound. For instance, if it calls for a light contact, press so lightly that there is little or no contact. And pay more attention to how the articulation of the word feels than how it sounds.

Although this post-block correction may seem to take a long time, it should not take over a few seconds. The more you do it and become adept at it, the less time it will take. The slow prolonged resonant way of working your way through the sound while keeping your voice flowing will give you plenty of time to feel yourself making the corrections you need to make.

---

[1]Move slowly and gently from sound to sound through the word. (Neely)

You need not be ashamed of repeating your stuttered words in this deliberate manner. The slight delay and the careful corrections will show others that you are determined to control your difficulty. Most listeners are considerate anyway, and they will actually respect you for your efforts.[1] You will need plenty of opportunity to use post-block corrections, and it may help some to practice them aloud when you are alone.

Obviously, duplicating a stuttering block can be a traumatic experience. And your tendency may be not to modify the block but rather to say the stuttered word a second time normally and rush onward as if nothing had happened. However, it should be pointed out that if you do so, you will miss the valuable benefit to be gained from this procedure.[2]

Persevere in using these corrections when you stutter. Their use will help you train yourself so you can move more easily through a block. They will break up the pattern of your stuttering and help you gain confidence in your ability to **control** your speech.

As one person expressed it, "this sounded easy but I found out a lot of time is necessary before you can count on saying the word the easy way." Another commented, "it was pretty tough to stutter and then wait to try again, but it's gotten easier. I learned more about my stuttering each time I did it."

---

[1] Most people, believe it or not, would be considerate and sympathetic of your problem. (Barbara)

[2] Do a good job on the post-block process of correction. This is where correction takes place. Don't just say the words over again fluently after you stutter. Say them carefully, concentrating on the feelings of muscular action as you coordinate the breath stream with the formation of sounds. Concentrate on the feelings of movement and fluence. (Starbuck)

K-k-k-katie, beautiful Katie
You're the only g-g-g-girl that I adore
And when the m-moon shines
Over the cowshed
I'll be waiting by the k-k-k-kitchen door.

Above are words from a favorite song published many years ago.
It would probably be more difficult to popularize such a song now.

Rule (8)

In-Block Correction

PULL-OUT

With the post-block correction, you learned how to cancel your stuttering after it had occurred. Now it is suggested that you can use a somewhat comparable method of pulling out of a block when you are in the midst of it.[1] This is to be used in those cases where you have the need for easing out of a block with which you are struggling.[2] What do you usually do when you feel yourself stuck in a block with no warning?

Perhaps you have tried to escape from such a block by using some intelligent procedure, but more probably you just struggle blindly, trying to force your way out. It would be better to use a systematic method, one that is compatible with this therapy approach, called an 'in-block' correction.

Here's the way it works. When you find yourself in the middle of a block, don't pause and don't stop and try again. Instead, continue the stuttering, slowing it down and letting the block run its course, deliberately making a smooth prolongation of what you are doing.[3] In doing this, you will

---

[1]You must learn how to pull out of your old blocks voluntarily, to get them under voluntary control before uttering the word. (Van Riper)

[2]It is possible to release yourself voluntarily from blocking or repeating prior to completing a word utterance. (Czuchna)

[3]He (the stutterer) can change the way he stutters by deliberately "hanging on to" or prolonging the troublesome sound without struggling or unnecessary forcing. (Luper)

be stabilizing the sound by slowing down a repetition, or changing the repetition to a prolongation, or smoothing out a tremor, or pulling out of a fixation as you ease out of the block.

In doing this, you will come to realize that you can control the duration of your block by changing the rate and then learning to smooth out your stutter.[1] Anyway, hold the stuttering long enough to feel control and figure out what you are doing wrong and what needs to be done to change your faulty actions. From your previous study, you should realize what you can do to counteract your incorrect speech behavior.

After you have figured this out, then voluntarily release yourself by discontinuing the prolongation or repetitions— and in slow motion put into effect the measures you decided would reverse or correct the abnormal speech muscle action.[2]

If for any reason you are unable to get hold of your stutter and move out of the block as described above, then it would be better for you to do a post-block correction in order for you to keep the feeling of being in control. In any case, you should be able to correct what you did wrong because of what you have learned from your analysis and study of the way you stutter.

---

[1] As stutterers learn that they can control the duration of the stuttering block, the fear of not being able to complete the message disappears. (D. Williams)

[2] In pulling out of blocks the stutterer does not let the original blocking run its course as he does in cancellation. Instead he makes a deliberate attempt to modify it before the release occurs and before the word is spoken. (Van Riper)

Pre-Block Correction

PREPARATORY SET

Presumably you have now conscientiously practiced and regularly employed post-block and in-block corrections when you stuttered. In doing this, you learned new ways of responding and how to move through a block in a predetermined manner. You should now be adept at correcting your stuttering after it happens.

However, you may have felt that post-block corrections were like locking the barn door after the horse was stolen since the process did not stop the stuttering when it started. Of course you are right, but it is essential for you to have had this training because it paves the way for this next step. Obviously, you now need to learn how to make preparations to forestall your stuttering before it happens.[1] This process of controlling your blocks before they occur is called 'pre-block' correction.

Most of the time, you anticipate when you may have trouble before it happens. In fact, stuttering is sometimes referred to as an "anticipatory struggle reaction," which in effect says that you anticipate trouble and react by struggling to avoid it. Occasionally there is no anticipation and the blocks surprise you. This will be discussed later.

---

[1]You must learn how to prepare for the speech attempt on feared words so they can be spoken without interference or abnormality. (Van Riper)

Since you usually have anticipation of difficulty before it happens, we propose that you take advantage of this fact. To do so will give you an opportunity to respond to the threat of trouble by preparing for it ahead of time.

So in this step, it is suggested that you learn how to cope with your stuttering by moving out ahead of a block and approaching it in a new and better way through employing a pre-block correction. This is similar to the post-block correction except for the fact that your planning is done before (pre) rather than after (post) the need arises.

In the pre-block correction, when you anticipate stuttering on a word or sound, you are to pause just before saying the word in order to plan how you will attack it. And you do not proceed to speak the word until you have thought about how you usually stutter on the sound and figure out what needs to be done to correct or modify the errors you usually make when stuttering on that sound.

Even though this course of action is similar to the post-block process, please study the following directions carefully so you will know exactly how it should be done. It is a key part of your therapy program.

To prevent any possible misunderstanding, we outline in detail how these pre-block corrections should be put into action. It will require concentration on your part. The numbers in parentheses refer to the steps in the procedure.

Pre-Block Correction—Sequence of Action

This is the exact procedure you should follow in using a pre-block correction when you approach a feared sound or word. Just as you come up to the word and before you start to say it, (1) pause—come to a complete stop. This pause before starting to say the word gives you time to calm yourself and to plan and rehearse how you will deal with the word.

The pause will not be long and a willingness to halt will convince both you as well as your listener that you are determined to be in control of the situation.[1] Even if it takes longer, the pause may be less embarrassing than your stuttering, particularly if you blunder into it blindly.

After you have stopped, (2) try to relax the tensed area of your speech mechanism including your throat. Try to get a feeling of your tongue lying limp in the bottom of your mouth with your jaw slightly open as if you were going to drool with your lips loose. See if you can get a feeling of looseness in that area.

As you relax, think back and (3) recall what you usually do abnormally when you block on that sound. What errors do you usually make when you stutter on it? You should remember these errors from the analysis and study you made of your speech muscle activity and from your experience in making post-block corrections.

Then from this review of the errors you usually make (4) figure out what corrections you learned to put into effect to change what you usually did wrong when you stuttered on that sound in order to help you eliminate or modify the abnormalities you make when you block on it.

Then (5) rehearse in your mind, or actually pantomime how it would feel in your mouth to put these corrections into

---

[1]Society in general rewards the person who obviously confronts and attempts to deal with his stuttering. (Stromsta)

effect, saying the whole word in a slow motion deliberately-prolonged manner, shifting slowly from one sound to the next. This means you are to mentally rehearse or pantomime how you will act out these changes to eliminate the errors you usually make on that sound.[1]

As your breathing returns to normal—and not before—(6) say the word, making the corrections as you rehearsed them. BUT (7) articulate the sound and word in a sliding resonant prolonged manner, exaggerating the corrections, paying more attention to how the word feels than how it sounds.[2] Although the slow articulation may carry over to the following few words, you should not talk that way otherwise.

A problem is often encountered in making the transition from the consonant sound to the vowel sound which follows. The slow prolonged manner of keeping the sounds flowing, as you utter the feared word, is designed to make that transition smooth.[3] Also it allows you sufficient time to get the feeling of making the corrections as you slide through the sound and word.[4] As you move slowly through the word, concentrate on getting the feel of change or overcorrecting your abnormalities.

---

[1]First, he (the stutterer) is to reduplicate in pantomime a fore-shortened version of the stuttering behavior he has just experienced and, secondly, he is to rehearse again in pantomime, a modified version of that behavior. (Van Riper)

[2]Learn to be aware of the feeling of muscle action as you move through a word. (Neely)

[3]Any action that emphasizes or enhances smooth transitions from sound to sound, syllable to syllable, or word to word, will be beneficial for on-going speech. (Agnello)

[4]These corrected words may seem prolonged and drawling. That happens as a result of the more careful and slower movements you made while saying the word. These will speed up as your skill improves. We are not after slow, drawling speech, but speech with more self-controlled movements. (Starbuck)

If you are embarrassed by the pause or by the drawling way you enunciate the feared word, do it anyway! This is where your determination pays off— you have no other choice. You will find that the pause will become shorter and shorter as you become more proficient at tackling your expected blocking in this new way.

> **Warning**—under no circumstances should you use the pause as a postponement, although it may be tempting to do so. The pause should be used to prepare and rehearse your plan of action.

This pre-block correction is an important part of your therapy program. If you can move smoothly through an anticipated block, you are well on your way to speaking freely and fluently. Practice pre-block corrections on both feared and nonfeared words—or on the first word of a sentence[1] but do not use them as a trick to get started. Some stutterers have pre-blocked on every word while they were learning the technique but that should not be necessary. The effect of a good pre-block carries over.

Select words on which you might block—figure out how you usually stutter on them—then determine what changes you need to make and apply them when you get to the word. Whenever you suspect trouble, put your controls into effect and pre-block. Continue this practice until you automatically feel what corrections are required for any type of block. This should give you the good feeling of knowing your stuttering is under control.

---

[1]It is always good to use a pre-block on the first word of a sentence. (Starbuck)

When you become so accustomed to using pre-block corrections that they are second nature to you, then you can start gradually eliminating the pause. When you anticipate trouble on a sound several words ahead, you can use the time during which you are saying the intervening words to prepare what you need to do when you reach the feared word.

Then put your speech into low gear (slow down) which will give you time to plan how you should make the necessary corrections. Then move slowly and smoothly through the word as you feel your way along.

This is your goal, and you may attain it fairly quickly, but until you have confidence in your ability to do it properly, it would be better for you first to stop and pause in order to allow yourself the time to make adequate preparations to deal with expected trouble.

As you get better at pre-block corrections, you will be building confidence in your ability to control your speech so you can move through any block in a predetermined manner. You determine beforehand the movements you have to make and how you have to make them to form the sounds and say the words smoothly. It is important to follow through on this. Stuttering is something you do, and you should now have learned how you can change what you have been doing.

Do You Get Discouraged?

If you are like many stutterers, sometimes you become quite discouraged while you are working on improving your speech. This could be because you are not getting better as quickly as you think you should, or because, on occasion, you relapse and have a lot of difficulty.

The latter may occur when you are speaking more easily and you run into a particularly embarrassing situation and tense up and fail miserably. This makes you quite despondent and undermines what confidence you may have built up that you are making progress.[1,2]

Unfortunately, stuttering seems to be particularly susceptible to reoccurring.[3] And it should be pointed out that there are several factors which are working against your efforts and which tend to cause or influence relapses or regression.

Relapses can occur because of natural tendencies to go back to using some of your old habits such as avoidances or denying your stuttering. You have begun to enjoy a certain amount of fluency; and to protect that fluency, your natural instincts influence you to react as you have been accustomed to doing for many years. Little facsimilies of your old stuttering habit may reappear.

---

[1]Every stutterer will have some ups and downs and the course of improvement is seldom a smooth course. (Kamhi)

[2]Despite progress there will be occasional days of poor talking for disorganizing stresses are sure to intervene. (Bluemel)

[3]The central problem of treatment is not the difficulty of bringing about fluency, but the high probability of relapse; few quick cures are likely to be durable; and in general the most reliable way to achieve a lasting reduction of stuttering is to do it slowly and gradually through a process that enlists the stutterers' comprehension of what they do when they stutter, why they do it, and how and why they are capable of altering their behavior. (Bloodstein)

There is no need to berate yourself when old habits recur. Still, when this happens you should recognize them as signals to get back on the job and review your compliance with the rules. And as you take care of these little avoidance feelings or any forcings, they will go away.

One factor which may contribute to frustration is the fact that almost every stutterer's severity tends to vary from time to time. Sometimes you speak more fluently than at other times. Although this may result from different environmental conditions, it seems that such deviations may persist, and therefore a breakdown is more easily triggered.

Another possible drawback to improvement sometimes occurs when your hopes are built up prematurely. This may be when some particular rule or guideline you adopted caused you to make such rapid improvement that you became convinced it was the answer to your problem. And if confidence in that particular procedure is lessened by failure, it tends to make the outlook more discouraging.

It is true that occasionally some one rule or corrective procedure may be a large part of the answer to your problem.[1] Generally, though, the application of the different procedures tends to assure more steady progress.[2]

---

[1] We are all different; what helps one stutterer may not work for another. (Garland)

[2] Fluency, like confidence comes slowly and slips back from time to time. (Guitar)

Another reason some people who stutter become discouraged is because they want and expect perfection which is unattainable. Some feel they should be able to talk perfectly with no hesitation or stumblings whatsoever. To expect perfection tends to build up pressure which they don't need. Normal speakers are not perfectly fluent, and your goal should be to work for easy speech with no strain.[1,2]

Besides, it is possible that you could have better natural coordination between that part of your brain that controls your speech and the timing sequence of your speech muscle action. That is also true of other people.

But there may be more reason for this being true in your case, particularly if your stuttering started when you were quite young. As a child, you may have had more hesitations or stumblings when learning to talk than other children. And some lack of better natural coordination mentioned above could have contributed to the development of your stuttering.

As you know, coordination is a physical attribute which varies with the individual. Just as some children learn to walk earlier than others, some learn to talk more easily than others. In adults, for instance, a champion golfer has superior coordination between that part of the brain which

---

[1]Don't waste your time and frustrate yourself by trying to speak with perfect fluency. (Sheehan)

[2]Lessen your demands on yourself and on others for perfect speech and total acceptance. (Barbara)

controls body movements and their action in guiding his golf clubs. In any case, a goal of perfection in speech is impractical for those who stutter.[1]

Most stutterers experience intervals of relative fluency filled with hope followed by episodes of blocking filled with despair. When relapse from fluency occurs, try to learn how to identify the source of the relapse. The answer should be somewhere in this book. Check your observance of the guidelines, and whenever you talk, don't force or struggle—stutter easily.

However, we would emphasize that there is no need to feel guilty every time you stutter—it doesn't mean that you are a failure. Most stutterers get discouraged at times. Stuttering is a tough enemy and needs to be beaten down time and time again into submission.[2] Accept this fact. Therapy may sometimes be an experience in frustration, but possibly you may be able to look on its experiences as having the possibility of revealing what might be done to achieve better speech.

With the high probability of relapse, it is difficult to bring about fluency quickly. It takes time. The most reliable way to bring about a lasting reduction of stuttering is to do it slowly and gradually.

Let's review the situation in the next chapter.

---

[1]Stutterers may be poorer than non-stutterers in coordinating the speech production processes. But despite being at the lower end of the normal distribution in coordinative ability, most stutterers are not so poor in these abilities that they cannot produce fluent speech. (Kamhi)

[2]It requires patience and a willingness to accept reoccurrences as well as remissions. (Garland)

Let's Review—What's Been Done

Let's review the situation and talk about what progress, if any, you have made. Possibly you have been reading this book just to learn more about stuttering and to find out how a therapy program works. If so, we hope you have enjoyed reading it. As a result, you should now have a better understanding of the ramifications of this complex problem.

But assuming you are a stutterer and have been honestly trying out the procedures outlined, you should have found out that you could change your speaking behavior by letting your speech be governed by the recommendations set by the ground rules.[1]

In starting to work this program, we presume you first sincerely experimented with the therapy procedure where you talked in a slow, sliding, prolonged manner which has alleviated the problem for some stutterers. If you used this slow, drawling manner of talking, it should have enabled you to communicate with less difficulty in situations where you might have had a lot of trouble. Although this method of talking probably helped you, we realize that normally you might not wish to talk that way all the time.[2]

Experimenting with that procedure should have shown whether or not you had the necessary determination to follow through on therapy procedures which would help you solve your problem. We hope you had that determination.[1]

---

[1]Stuttering behavior can be changed. Even though you may have no choice as to whether or not you stutter, you do have a choice of how you stutter. (Murray)

[2]Alleviating one's stuttering is ultimately a matter of self-discipline and control. (Stromsta)

Then, supposedly you proceeded to work on the ground rules. It would be too much to expect completely satisfactory observance with all their objectives. But if you followed these guidelines, you have found that you can control your difficulty, partly through modifying your feelings and attitudes toward your stuttering— and partly through modifying the abnormal actions associated with your stuttering behavior.

Okay, you started on the rules. In complying with some of them, you were not told to stop your stuttering but were asked to make certain calming changes in your manner of talking.

For instance, you were first (1) urged to make a habit of talking slowly and deliberately. Then, even more importantly, (2) you were asked to stutter easily, gently and smoothly, prolonging the starting sounds of feared words and the transition to the next sounds. Also, it was suggested (10) that you try to vary your speech rate and loudness and speak with expression in a melodious manner.

All right, what happened? Do you now make a habit of always talking in a slow and deliberate manner? And do you make a point of stuttering easily, gently and smoothly— in as expressive and melodious a manner as possible? If you complied with these requests, you are talking with less tension and the frequency, and severity of your difficulty must have lessened. That means you have made some progress.

But you still stutter. Then, to cut down on the fear of difficulty you experience you were asked to change certain habits which reinforced that fear. In one rule (3) you were told to quit trying to hide the fact that you were a stutterer—in fact openly admit that you were one. But even more importantly (5) you were to stop all avoidance, substitution or postponement habits you used to get around expected trouble. That was a tough one, too. And likewise (6) you were told to continually maintain good, natural eye contact when stuttering to help reduce feelings of shame.

Have you definitely changed your attitude and conduct so that you will now openly discuss your stuttering with anybody? Also, do you maintain good eye contact with your listener when having difficulty? And can it be assumed that you no longer try to avoid, postpone or substitute? If you have complied with these rules, you have eliminated much of the worry and anxiety which torments stutterers and increases their tension. Just to have decreased some of your fears should have made life more pleasant.

All of the above was primarily essential in helping you calm some of the tension and reduce some of the fears which are the basic ingredients causing or aggravating your trouble.

Under (4) you worked on finding out if you had any secondary symptoms accompanying your stuttering. And if you did, supposedly you worked to eliminate them—so hopefully, you are now rid of that part of your stuttering act. Accordingly, your stuttering was then confined to irregularities in the way you operated your speech mechanism.

Your next step under rule (7) was to make a careful study of your stuttering pattern. To do this, it was necessary to accurately duplicate what you had your speech mechanisms do when you stuttered. Accordingly, by monitoring your speech you obtained a clear understanding of what you did irregularly or abnormally with your speech muscles (lips, tongue and jaw) which was not needed in the production of speech.

Having obtained this valuable detailed information about your wrong speech muscle actions, you were asked to modify or eliminate these by employing block corrections. These key procedures (8) were not easy to work but were organized to eliminate or modify the articulatory errors which you made when stuttering.

They were designed to help you guide your speech muscle movements easily and smoothly into, through and out of your blocks by substituting new patterns for old habits. These procedures should have helped you to modify the irregular actions which characterized your stutter.

Theoretically this eliminated your stuttering; but practically, it should have at least helped you to speak without much or all of the blocking maneuvers you previously experienced—habits which you now know can be unlearned.

The other rules not mentioned above were part of your program and we assume were not overlooked. One of them (9) urged that you keep your speech moving forward with no repetitions or back-tracking so as to keep continuous voicing progress.

Another (11) advocated that you pay more attention and think more about what fluency you had. You have worried about and brooded over your stuttering long enough. And if you have made a point of feeling what fluency you have, the more it should have helped you to build confidence. And obviously, it is presumed (12) that you have tried to talk as much as possible as otherwise you would not have made the opportunities you needed to work on your speech.

The above briefly summarizes the results which we hope you were able to accomplish in following the twelve rules or guidelines. Have you given it time? Where are you now? See next chapter for conclusions.

Where Are You—Conclusion

If you have done your best to comply with all these guidelines, you have completed this therapy program. We don't know how fluent you have become—possibly you have come a long way—possibly you haven't. This book only describes an approach which will work. You are the one who has produced the results.[1]

In following this program, you now more willingly admit that you stutter and hopefully you continue to eliminate any avoidance habits you may have had. This should have helped relieve a lot of your anxiety and helped you develop more self-confidence as well as increased your ability to tolerate stress.

Also if you have learned nothing else, you should have found out that you can change your way of talking.[2,3] And if you can vary the pattern of your stuttering, you can learn to control it. You want and need that feeling of control which enables you to talk easily and comfortably.

And if you had the patience to stick to your guns in this program, we'll bet you're glad that you didn't back out. But even for those who have made rapid progress, we advise caution. Strange as it may seem you may need to adjust to fluent speech.[4]

---

[1]It is not a matter of luck. You can make your own "luck." You can get there. (J. D. Williams)

[2]Speech is something produced by the speaker and as such is something the speaker can modify and change. (Conture)

[3]By learning that he has a choice in the way he talks and in the manner in which he reacts, he will come to realize that he can be responsible for the way he talks. He will come to be the kind of speaker who can change the speaking he does. (D. Williams)

[4]You may be astonished that fluency is anything to which you would have to adjust. Yet it is a central problem in the consolidation of improvement. (Sheehan)

You may need to monitor your speech as you become fluent, depending on your reactions. For instance, you may start talking so fast that you do not become aware of avoidances or struggles that could develop. Furthermore, since you have not been accustomed to talking freely, any inability to express yourself in managing phrases or sentences may cause you to lose confidence in your way of talking.[1]

As has been pointed out, unfortunately, stuttering seems to be particularly susceptible to reoccurring.[2] You will need to guard against slipping back into old habits. Habits which you acquired years ago and which have been performed for many years can reinstate themselves if you aren't careful. You may at times be confronted with old fears.

If you are confronted with such fears, the most important point for you to remember is that a **willingness to stutter in a modified way** can be a tremendous help in sustaining and reinforcing your fluency.

Also to help prevent backsliding or regression, do your best to make certain that your speech is governed the ground rules. These common sense measures can always help you communicate with less stress and strain. And be sure that you do not start avoiding.

---

[1] We have seen stutterers who have become quite fluent following therapy, but who still lack conversational skills. A typical example would be the young man who is no longer afraid to talk to a young woman, but who doesn't know what to say when he meets one. (Guitar-Peters)

[2] Traces of the disorder usually remain and relapses occur. (Freund)

If you run into any unusual difficulty, you can always use block corrections. It might be well to review and practice them occasionally anyway since you may always be able to use them to advantage.

Actually as time passes on, you should continue to gain confidence in your ability to control your speech.[1] Be assertive; the more confidence you have, the more freedom from fear you will experience.

It will help if you adopt a positive attitude generally. Tell yourself that you can and will overcome your difficulty. If you can adopt an assertive attitude and combine it with controlled techniques, you will improve faster.

Believe in yourself, be assertive, and have confidence in your endeavors.

On the other hand don't expect or claim too much.[2] Don't be too anxious to talk too well too soon and don't make excessive demands on your speech which will be impossible to achieve. And don't be fooled into thinking that just because you don't stutter that that automatically makes you witty, charming and persuasive.[3]

If someone says you are cured, don't feel that you have to prove it. Instead tell him or her that you still stutter and actually show them that you can do so by stuttering voluntarily. If you always call yourself a stutterer, you will be under no pressure not to be one. Remember stuttering is largely what you do trying not to stutter.

---

[1] Confidence comes when we do battle and succeed. It comes when we accept a challenge instead of running away from it. (Van Riper)

[2] On the whole people who stutter are highly intelligent and capable. Yet there appears to be a discrepancy between their realistic capabilities and potentialities and what they realistically expect of themselves....To avoid this dilemma, make your expectations more reasonable. (Barbara)

[3] Stutterers are no better or no worse than anyone else, and you would not necessarily set the world on fire if you only did not stutter. You would just talk better. (Emerick)

Your speech, like that of others, doesn't have to be perfect.[1] Most people are disfluent and don't have verbal perfection—stutterers or not. Stuttering is a stubborn handicap and if you have conquered it to the extent that you have freedom from fear, you can no longer claim it as a handicap.[2] Therapy is a challenge as life is a challenge. Have faith in yourself.[3]

And if you have just been reading this book for information, we would again point out that there is no reason for you to spend the rest of your life stuttering helplessly and making yourself miserable.

Others have prevailed and so can you. Program yourself for success and have confidence in your ability to achieve it.

The End

---

[1]Perfect fluency is not obtainable and is a self-defeating goal. (Sheehan)

[2]If the fear of stuttering can be reduced, then certainly stuttering itself can be reduced. (Rainey)

[3]After all, fellow stutterers, there are strength and resources within each of us. Only through these can we really accomplish anything. (Brown)

A Personal Letter to You

Smile and make up your mind that you are going to be happier and get more joy out of life!

As you follow the suggestions in this book, bear in mind that stuttering is your problem and yours alone, and it probably will take a lot of discipline and desire to accomplish your purpose.

Adopt a positive attitude, and encourage yourself to maintain a realistic commitment to undertake the difficult assignments needed for progress.

And since you may have been stuttering for years, it may take time to achieve the success you are looking for— but it can be done, and the result is worth the trouble.

Here's wishing you freedom from fear and a happier life.

Sincerely yours,

Malcolm Fraser

Life's battles don't always go
   To the strongest or fastest man;
But sooner or later the man who wins
   Is the man who thinks he can!

Information—Appendix

Sharing Problems with Others

Self-help or support groups have been organized in many places across the country. At their regularly scheduled meetings, those who stutter have the opportunity to discuss their problem with others who are having the same difficulty. Some meetings are organized by speech clinicians in conjunction with university or college speech pathology departments.

At such group meetings, it is comforting to talk over and share experiences with others who are sympathetic and understanding because they have been though the same trouble. Counseling with others, including the use of speech in social situations, should help you.[1]

These meetings are an ideal place to work on emphasizing the desirable modification procedures designed to help you become a better communicator. Talking in front of a group helps to build self confidence, something which is badly needed by all who stutter. Participating in such a group may help you develop a better insight and understanding of how others react to their communicator. When the group has the right sort of leadership, we urge their support. It also gives one the opportunity to reach out and help others with the same difficulty.

---

[1]Common sharing of feelings is one of the hallmarks of these self-help groups and this is very therapeutic. (Gregory)

Explaining to a Non-Stutterer the Effect of Fear

If you should have occasion to explain to a non-stutterer how fear of difficulty can affect one's speech, the following illustration could be used. Assuming the non-stutterer has nothing wrong with his legs, you could point out that probably he could walk easily without trouble or quite "fluently" along a long plank, twelve inches wide, when it is placed on the ground.

But if that same plank is placed on a wall high above the ground, then, if asked to walk along the plank, he would probably develop a fear of falling. As a result, it would be difficult for him to walk along the plank in a normal way. In fact he would probably put on a poor exhibition of walking normally or "fluently."

This example is somewhat parallel to the problem of stuttering. Nearly all stutterers have the physical equipment to talk properly, but in many cases the fear of stuttering causes them to try to force trouble-free speech. And since it is difficult to force the articulative mechanism of speech, he does not speak fluently.

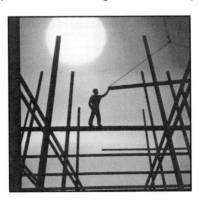

On Breath Control

Although easy, quiet breathing is helpful in enabling the stutterer to speak more freely, it is not suggested that the stutterer try to consciously control the inhalation and exhalation of his breath. Trying to consciously control breath can too often result in breathing abnormalities including speaking at the end of breath, gasping or hyperventilation with a resulting increase in tension.[1]

When the stutterer speaks slowly and smoothly, particularly in the initiation of words, in an easy onset manner with soft contacts, it will help to influence natural and proper breathing.

In an effort to eliminate stuttering, some speech pathologists recommend that the stutterer should make a slight "sigh" as he tackles a block with the thought that this would keep his vocal cords open and relaxed which would enable him to move more easily through the block. This is somewhat similar to the recommendation that a stutterer make or breathe a silent "h" sound when starting to say a feared word.

Such techniques can work, as they will help release tension in the vocal cords because they distract the mind from fear. However, as such distractive effect wears off, the stutterer may be left with abnormalities such as mentioned above.

To sum it up, it takes very little breath to speak. So since breathing is more or less automatic, it should usually not be necessary for a stutterer to try to keep it under conscious control.[2]

---

[1]There are dangers in the deliberate control of the breath for speaking. (Van Riper)

[2]Breath control is best when it is automatic and not under conscious control....Breathing should be relatively automatic and unconscious so, in general, the less attention you give to it, the better. (Luper)

Electronic Devices Used in Conjunction With Stuttering Treatment

Electronic aids and other devices have been around for many years. Some people who stutter have found them to be helpful, at least in limited situations such as on the telephone or when giving a speech. Others who may have hoped for a "magic cure" have been disappointed because the devices can be cumbersome and make conversation difficult.

Our advice, before you spend a considerable sum of money on an electronic aid for stuttering, is to consult with qualified speech-language pathologists who have experience in prescribing and fitting the aid.

If possible, you may also want to log on to a discussion group of individuals who stutter and parents of children who stutter where you can ask for advice and feedback about using such a device. Such a forum should provide you with relatively unbiased testimony from those who have tried these aids and found them helpful, or, in some cases, not helpful.

You may call the Stuttering Foundation at 800-992-9392 for a list of electronic aids or see them listed at www.stutteringhelp.org.

Some Tips On Using the Phone

Many people—whether they stutter or not—have difficulty using the telephone.

Listen to some non-stutterers dealing with phone calls. Some take several seconds to answer. Others may "Um" and "Ah" a lot. Others may be very expressive with their hands or faces, perhaps talking loudly and aggressively.

If, as a person who stutters, you have a problem using the telephone, then you may find the following advice helpful. Using the phone can cause a great deal of anguish, and each person must learn to cope with it in his or her own way.

Making Calls To Others

Making a call can usually be split into three phases: preparation, the call, assessing how you did.

■ Preparation

Make sure you know why you are calling. Write the key points on paper and have it in front of you when you call.

Try phoning a friend or relative just before the big call. This may help relax you.

If you have a number of calls to make, list them in ascending order. Start with the easiest and work your way up to the most difficult.

Do not keep putting off the call you need to make. That will make it even more stressful and difficult.

■ The Call

Quite often the difficult part is getting through to the right person. If you are confronted by a switchboard operator, for example, would an extension number or department be easier to say than someone's name? Have some alternative first words in mind; be flexible in what you want to say. If you do start to block, stutter openly, gently and easily; try not to force the words out and most importantly remember to speak slowly.

Do not worry too much about silences; they occur in all conversations. Concentrate on what you have to say, rather than worry about any blocks. Your purpose is to communicate, whether you stutter or not. Pay attention to your fluent speech. Many stutterers forget about their times of fluency and dwell on the stuttering. Savor your fluency; make other calls when feeling more fluent; strike while the iron is hot. Fluent speech breeds confidence, and confidence breeds fluent speech.

Watching yourself in a mirror while phoning can be helpful as you will be able to see where the tension lies in your face and other parts of your body. If you persevered with a difficult call and felt you communicated well, then praise or treat yourself and remember the good feeling that a successful call gave you.

■ Assessing How You Did

Most people, not just those who stutter, sometimes make calls when they feel they have been less than fluent or have not managed to get their message across.

If you felt that a particular call was stressful and you stuttered more than usual, try to forget it. Adopt a positive attitude; remember there will be other conversations when you will stutter less. It is not a disaster to stutter, and you can learn from each speaking experience. At home, tape-record your telephone conversations if you can. Note your speech carefully, especially the speed and the lead up to any blocks. Try to learn from each recording, and prepare a strategy for the next call. Doing this over a period of time will help to identify certain recurring problems and words.

Receiving Calls

This is the area over which you have least control. However, even here you can go part way to easing some of the pressure you may feel. Always answer the call in your own time. Don't rush to the telephone. Again have key word options ready: your extension number, name of your organization, or even just your name. Use whatever comes easiest to you at that moment.

If you receive a call within earshot of other people, concentrate solely on that call.

Accept that others may hear and see you block, but do not allow their presence to distract you from your phone call.

Don't be afraid of initial silence on the phone if you struggle for your first word. It is quite common for someone to answer the phone and then not speak, either because they're finishing a conversation with a colleague or because they have picked up someone else's phone and are waiting for them to return to their seat.

The person phoning you may also stutter. Be patient with others who may be just as anxious as you and may be putting into practice some of the above points.

Eliminating Stereotypes About Stuttering

- People who stutter are as intelligent and well-adjusted as those who don't.

- Don't assume that people who stutter are prone to be nervous, anxious, fearful, or shy. While stuttering behaviors may sometimes resemble the behaviors of those who experience these emotions, people who stutter exhibit the same full range of personality traits as those who do not.

- Stuttering is not the result of emotional conflict or fearfulness.

- People who stutter often have excellent communications skills. They should not be seen as deficient at verbal communication. Some are very often qualified for and interested in positions requiring them to deal with members of the public on a daily basis.

- People who stutter have the same ambitions and goals for advancement as non-stutterers. To an extent consistent with their abilities, they should be offered leadership opportunities and paths for promotion within an organization.

- Stuttering varies widely in different people and varies in the same person over different times and places. People who stutter often have "good" and "bad" days with their speech.

- For people who stutter, a job interview is perhaps the single most difficult speaking situation they will ever encounter and is not indicative of how they would speak on the job. It is important to consider the actual job requirements and conditions.

This information is from the brochure Answers for Employers, *which can be downloaded at www.stutteringhelp.org, click on "Brochures for all ages." This brochure is perfect for job interviews.*

Relevant Questions and Interesting Quotations

How many people stutter?

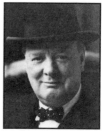

Winston Churchill

Few realize that almost one percent of the population stutter, that there are more than three million stutterers in the United States today. That many famous people from history have had essentially the same problem, including Moses, Demosthenes, Charles Lamb, Charles Darwin, and Charles I of England. More recently George VI of England, Winston Churchill, Somerset Maugham, Marilyn Monroe, and the television personalities, Garry Moore and Jack Paar have been stutterers at some time in their lives. In your speech problem you may not be as unique or as much alone as you had thought! (Sheehan)

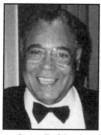

James Earl Jones

The incidence of stuttering amounts to about 3,000,000 in this country alone. It has been placed at about one percent of the general population, roughly half of them are children. Stuttering has no respect for social or economic status, religion, race or intelligence.

Is there a Web site where I can download information on stuttering?

The Stuttering Foundation's Web sites, www.stutteringhelp.org and www.tartamudez.org, contain information for the general public as well as specific help for those who stutter and their families. This online source is proving an extremely useful tool in raising awareness about stuttering, dispelling common myths, and providing helpful resources.

Is anything being done to increase public awareness of stuttering?

The following nationally-recognized spokespersons have worked with the Stuttering Foundation to promote National Stuttering Awareness Week.

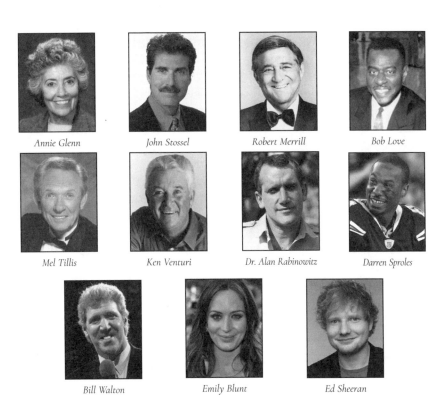

Annie Glenn   John Stossel   Robert Merrill   Bob Love

Mel Tillis   Ken Venturi   Dr. Alan Rabinowitz   Darren Sproles

Bill Walton   Emily Blunt   Ed Sheeran

Does stuttering tend to come and go?

Stuttering is intermittent. Even severe stutterers often speak more words normally than in stuttered fashion. The intermittency, however, makes the experience more distressful, since it is difficult to adapt to unpleasantness which comes and goes. (Van Riper)

When is stuttering apt to get worse?

When your morale or ego strength is high because of achievements, success or social acceptance, you will tend to stutter less. If in any given communicative situation you expect or feel communicative stress, penalties and frustrations, you will stutter more.

You will stutter more if you are experiencing or anticipating anxiety, guilt and hostility. You will also stutter more if in scanning ahead you see words or situations coming which have been associated with past experiences of stuttering.

Those who stutter have more trouble talking to authority figures, to people who have become impatient or mock or suffer when listening to stuttering. Most are very vulnerable to listener loss, to interruptions, to rejections, penalty, frustration, anxiety and hostility.

The pressures then, which create more stuttering can come from within or without, from the pressures of the present, the expected agonies of the future or the miseries of the past. (Van Riper)

Why are you apt to have difficulty saying your name?

It is especially hard for someone who stutters to say his name, as there is not only the problem of having to speak the name usually quickly, but one's name carries a heavy self-concept psychological load. It identifies one. It represents the whole person—all of his ideas that others have about him as well as his own self-concepts.

In addition, there is virtually no possibility of substituting another name for one's own name. Of all the words in a person's vocabulary, our name is representative of something we should know and utter with unhesitating automaticity. To do otherwise implies all sorts of possibilities, none of them associated with normality. Since most stutterers have innumerable failures trying to say their own names, their names as cue words acquire immense compulsive force. (Murray)

Should you work to be less sensitive?

During my first two years in college I began to see more clearly that a stutterer has to take responsibility for making others feel comfortable in his presence. If he can be less sensitive about his stuttering, those around him will be more comfortable. This will make him more at ease, and he will stutter less, and so it goes; the vicious circle will be put into reverse. Since I was doing something constructive about my speech, I could smile about difficulty more. I could even feign some voluntary disfluency. (Gregory)

Should you face up to fear?

My youth, as is the case with so many stutterers, was filled with alternate hope and despair as I hungered for some relief from my stuttering. This of course is not unique; most stutterers have had similar feelings. But have you ever asked yourself what it is that really bothers you, what it is that causes despair? Is it your stuttering or is it your fear of people's reactions to your stuttering? Isn't it the latter? Most stutterers have too much anxiety about what they think people might say or do as a result of the stuttering.

These anxieties can be lessened.

I remember well these feelings of worry, anxiety, and despair. If you can learn to dissipate some of these terrible feelings—you will be able to help yourself as many other stutterers have done.

There is one effective method you can utilize to achieve this goal. Face your fears! This advice is easy to give and admittedly difficult for many of you to take; however, it is advice that has helped many stutterers and it can help you.

Somehow you must learn to desensitize yourself to the reactions of others and refuse to let people's actual or imagined responses to your stuttering continue to affect your mental health or your peace of mind. (Adler)

Can you be temporarily helped by practically any type of treatment?

The fact is that stutterers may be helped for some time by practically any type of therapy in which they believe strongly has some important implications. It means that they may be especially likely to obtain short-term benefit from a therapist who is deeply convinced of the effectiveness of the methods used, who happens to be endowed with charisma and who has a prestigious role (e.g. physician, psychiatrist or the like). (Bloodstein)

Why is it hard to pause?

Many stutterers show a *fear of silence* and any momentary pause or cessation of sound in their own speech brings on reactions approaching panic. Perhaps because most stuttering occurs on initial syllables and the stutterer has more trouble when he starts, he learns to dread the necessity for starting. He learns to dread any period of silence in his own speech, to fear it, and to become quite intolerant of it. (Sheehan)

Should you take responsibility for your problem?

I also found, in working on my speech, that one makes many discoveries that can be applied advantageously to daily living. From the time I began therapy I have realized that I must take responsibility for my behavior and the way in which others evaluate me. In addition, I became aware of the tendency to lean on my stuttering as an excuse for not participating in some activity or for not being as successful as I might strive to be. (Gregory)

How severe can a block be?

The writer was a student at Stanford University and came home for a two week vacation and at that time was stuttering badly. As he tells it: "One afternoon I was studying in my room, writing with an ink pen. I accidentally knocked the ink bottle over, and ink spilled over my papers, my book, the fresh blotter, the wood of the desk, and down onto the rug beneath. My mother, sitting in the next room, heard my gasp and called to me asking what had happened. I went to the door of her room, and, as I stood there, trying to answer, I felt as though someone had grabbed me by the shoulders and was shaking me violently. My face, twisted with my struggle to break the tremor, turned red and then purple. I felt as though a gigantic balloon were stretching bigger and bigger, about to burst with a devastating force, and I had no way to protect myself from it. Just then the word 'ink!' exploded out of me. That was the worst block I have ever experienced. It must have been forty or fifty seconds long." (Murray)

Has rhythmic beat been used extensively in the treatment of stuttering?

In his younger days, the author attended several of these commercial stammering institutes and, from what he has read, they were typical of most of the others that exploited stutterers in the early years of the century....One used arm swinging, another the swaying of eyes or hands or body, the third a lalling rhythmic form of continuous utterance in which all words were joined and all consonants were slurred. (Van Riper)

What kind of job should I look for?

On the whole, people who stutter are highly intelligent and capable. Yet there appears to be a discrepancy between their realistic capacities and potentialities and what they unrealistically expect of themselves. Although there are many areas of productivity through which an individual can express his capacities and earn a comfortable living, I have

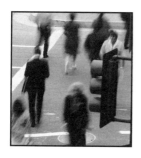

found that many people who stutter seem to be drawn toward jobs or professions where the use of verbal communication is paramount. It is not uncommon to find people who have difficulty speaking becoming salesmen, lawyers, psychologists, and radio announcers. (Barbara) *Editor's note: Download the brochure* Answers for Employers *at www.stutteringhelp.org for more information.*

Isn't it better to substitute words which are easier said?

You will feel better about your speech if you reduce the number of times you substitute non-feared words for feared ones. To test this out make five telephone calls and keep an account of the number of times you substituted non-feared words for feared ones. Then make five more telephone calls in which you try to make as few substitutions as possible. You should feel better about your speech when you are not substituting words or switching phrases to avoid stuttering. You may find that your **fear of stuttering** is actually *more* of a problem than your stuttering. (Trotter)

Shouldn't you just avoid trouble when speaking?

Above all, keep in mind that the less you struggle in your efforts not to stutter, and the less you avoid feared words and situations, *the less you will stutter in the long run.* (J. D. Williams)

In his efforts to speak fluently, the stutterer becomes more and more fearful of being unable to cope with the intermittent stuttering that may occur. The more he struggles to avoid possible stuttering or attempts to hide or disguise his stuttering that cannot be avoided, the more he denies that he has a problem. (Czuchna)

The only disability some people still laugh at.

Perhaps the day shall come when I can completely forgive those who have ridiculed and imitated my stuttering. As yet I have failed to find any more excuse for this than laughing at the crippled or the blind. I believe that those who torment the stutterer do so to compensate for some weakness or shortcoming of their own. (Wedberg)

Working on introducing yourself.

Between the ages of fifteen and twenty I worked rather intensely on my speech and gradually realized that I would need to work on situations of increasing difficulty by planning, experiencing and then planning again, etc., until I became more and more confident. For example, during my freshman year in college I worked on intro- 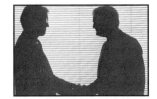 ducing myself. After working to keep eye contact with my listener, I worked on modifying my speech and using some voluntary disfluency when saying "I'm Hugo Gre-Gregory." By the end of the year I never avoided introducing myself or making introductions. (Gregory)

Shouldn't you try for perfect fluency?

Normal speech contains disfluencies of many types. (Moses)

It is good for you to realize that much of your own hesitating and fumbling in speaking is like that of other folks. If you are like other speakers who think of themselves as stutterers, you tend to suppose that unless your speech flows as smoothly as a meadow brook, you are not talking normally. Actually, many of your disfluencies are like those of normal speakers and are so regarded by them when they hear you. (Johnson)

A perfect flow of language formulation and speech production is a rare skill. Most of us have errors in formulation and imperfections in our speech produc- tion....Compare what you do with what your

friends do. They also repeat sounds, words and phrases, interject "uh" or stop while saying a difficult word. Therapy should lead toward acceptable, free flowing speech but not *perfect fluency.* (Boehmler)

The stutterer has a Demosthenes* complex. He makes demands on his speech and intellect which are excessive and impossible to achieve. This verbal perfectionism creates inner chaos and turmoil. The person who tends toward stut- tering feels that he should always speak calmly, *never* appear ruffled and *constantly* be in control of his listener. When he speaks he demands of himself the ultimate and impossible. He feels he should be the master of his words and have a reservoir of everflowing facts and ideas. He should speak in a clear and concise manner, pause at the right time, and never run ahead of his ideas and be contin- ually spontaneous when talking....To avoid this dilemma *make your expectations more reasonable.* (Barbara)

*Demosthenes lived in the fourth century B.C. and is considered one of the greatest orators of all time. He was such a powerful speaker that his orations rallied the citizens of Athens to oppose and defeat Alexander the Great, which significantly affected the history of ancient Greece. Supposedly, he overcame a speech defect (stuttering?) by stand- ing on the seashore with pebbles under his tongue and shouting above the roar of the waves.

Maybe Demosthenes had the right idea?

Growing up as a severe stutterer, I would hear such stories almost daily, starting with the legend of Demosthenes' pebbles. After trying everything else, I did attempt to talk with pebbles myself once. I didn't quite believe the legend, but I felt I should leave no stones untried. I almost swallowed the pebbles and quickly resumed the search for new crutches. (Sheehan)

Should you beware of following everybody's advice?

Stuttering is a disorder which can be worsened by ill treatment. Many well-meaning but ignorant individuals, by their suggestions and reactions, have made the stuttering not only more difficult to bear but also more severe and frequent. As in all speech disorders, this one needs special understanding. (Van Riper)

For years most adults who stutter have received well meaning suggestions that have been directly or indirectly aimed at stopping the stuttering altogether. These suggestions imply miraculously quick cures and fluent speech.

Every stutterer grows up with the naive advice of neighbors and casual strangers ringing uselessly in his ears. "Relax, think what you have to say, slow down, take a deep breath, did you ever try to talk with pebbles in your mouth, etc., etc."

Stuttering is a complex problem whose nature forever tempts people to offer simplistic cures. Neighbors and casual acquaintances usually do not offer advice on treating cancer or diabetes. But stuttering has a persistence along with a now-you-see-it-now-you-don't quality, so it fosters irresponsible and/or fraudulent claims for every solution. Simplistic "cures" abound, and the history of medicine is littered with them. Even intelligent people who should know better are taken in, and ensnare themselves. (Sheehan)

Should you explain stuttering to others?

Sometimes it is helpful to explain something about your stuttering to people who are important to you. This person might be a parent, teacher, friend, employer or a fellow worker. You might explain, for example, how you like to be treated by your listener when you are stuttering. The purpose of this is to make you and the people you speak with more relaxed concerning your stuttering. If you feel that a person understands your stuttering, you are likely to stutter less to that person. An open and honest attitude is healthy for all people involved. (Trotter)

A reason to become a "professional stutterer."

At about this time I began my training as a speech pathologist and embarked upon a career, as my wife and children tell friends, of being a "professional stutterer." By the way, I've always noticed that when my wife tells some person "Hugo is a professional stutterer," the person looks somewhat perplexed as if to say, "Does he stutter?" or, "Why do you mention it?" The point is we should be **very open about our stuttering**. I found out very early that this attitude is an important ingredient in therapy. (Gregory)

Can you change?

"The leopard can't change his spots." If you are in the habit of thinking and saying things like that, you are likely to tell yourself also "once a stutterer always a stutterer"— you might then go on to the depressing thought that there's really no hope for you.

Or if there is, there is the wishful hope that somewhere sometime you will be lucky and find someone who will take away, or drive away, what you *have* and transform you, as though by sorcery, from the stutterer you are into the normal speaker you long to be one day.

Such wishfulness makes for dreams, particularly daydreams, about magical potions in the form of pills, or secret or mysterious methods that can work wonders. It does not encourage you to face up to the problem yourself and do something constructive about it here and now by your own efforts.

What you have learned to do that keeps you from speaking better than you do, you can unlearn. (Johnson)

Does recovery take long?
Recovery is going to be a long gradual process. (Murray)

If the stutterer is going to change radically his accustomed manner of stuttering, he must work persistently and diligently over a long period of time. (Johnson)

Licking the problem of stuttering, mastering your own mouth, takes time; it cannot be accomplished overnight. How long will it take you I cannot say, for no two stutterers approach the challenge in the same way or move at the same rate but all have in common a beckoning mirage luring them ahead. (Emerick)

A memorable experience.
One score and seven years ago, in a desperate attempt to cure their son's chronic speech problem, my parents spent their meager savings to send me to a commercial school for stammering. Alas, to their dismay and my deepening feeling of hopelessness, it was just another futile attempt. While I rode woefully toward home on the train, a kindly old gray-haired conductor stopped at my seat and asked my destination. I opened my mouth for the well-rehearsed "Detroit" but all that emerged was a series of muted gurgles; I pulled my abdominal muscles in hard to break the terrifying constriction in my throat—silence. Finally, the old man peered at me through his bifocals, shook his head, and with just the trace of a smile, said, "Well, young man, either express yourself or go by freight."

The conductor had shuffled on down the aisle of the rocking passenger car before the shock waves swept over me. Looking out the window at the speeding landscape through a tearful mist of anger and frustration, I felt the surreptitious glances of passengers seated nearby; a flush of crimson embarrassment crept slowly up my neck and my head throbbed with despair. Long afterwards I remembered the conductor's penetrating comment. For years I licked that and other stuttering wounds and nursed my wrath to keep it warm, dreaming that someday I would right all those unrightable wrongs. But in the end his pithy pun changed my life. The old man, incredibly, had been right. (Emerick)

How well did King George VI of England speak in his radio broadcasts?

One of the people whose activities I followed closely was King George VI of England. I tuned in to his first Christmas broadcast with considerable excitement, because I had heard

King George VI

that he was a stutterer. Even though pre-recording was beginning to be available in those days, he had chosen to make his speech a live one.

I got the BBC at the right time and heard, through the static, "Ladies and Gentlemen, His Majesty, King George VI." He started without difficulty, but then his speech began to be more and more labored. He paused between words, first briefly and then the spaces grew longer. I could sense from the rhythms that a block was coming; and I held my breath waiting for it. There was one long silence, brief sounds of vocal struggle, and then quick repetitions out of which burst the word. This happened several times during that early broadcast.

In spite of his impediment, King George continued to speak publicly. He inspired his country when it needed him most. I heard him declare war on Germany. He was so emotional he could hardly speak, and yet his message was clear.

Although he was never completely free of all traces of stuttering, King George's speech improved enormously during his reign. His speeches were carefully pruned so that he wouldn't have to say words that usually caused him to block. His final illness began to sap his strength, and he stuttered considerably in his Christmas broadcast that year. (Murray)

About how much would it cost to engage the services of a professional speech therapist—a specialist in stuttering—to help you work on your speech?

Therapy charges can vary by geographic area and also the therapist's level of skill/specialization in working with a particular population. Private practitioners charge from $60 to $150 per hour. Most often the fee will be $70 to $85 an hour. Total cost could be from one to several thousand dollars.

Of course, in the case of short term treatment such as that described for some children beginning to stutter, it could be less. University clinics where students are being trained or publicly supported institutions charge on a sliding scale according to ability to pay, and the therapy will be less expensive. For example, the range might be from $20 to $80 an hour.

You should be satisfied with progress as therapy proceeds and feel free to inquire about the prognosis and costs. Health insurance policy coverage of stuttering therapy varies. If insurance reimburses for therapy, expect to pay a co-payment similar to what you would pay for other specialists such as physical therapists. You should consult with your agent and request that the speech clinician send reports or any other required information to the company.

For more information on how to find a therapist and on how to deal with insurance claims, call the Stuttering Foundation toll free number, 800-992-9392, or visit www.stutteringhelp.org.

Boyhood recollections...

What I remember most acutely about my stuttering is not the strangled sound of my own voice, but the impatient looks on other people's faces when I had trouble getting a word out. And if their eyes happened to reflect some of the pain and frustration I was feeling, that only made me more uneasy. There was nothing they could do to help me, and I certainly didn't want their sympathy. I was nine or ten at the time.

Like most people with a stuttering problem, I had already learned to live by my wits in a way that normally fluent people cannot begin to appreciate. Whenever I opened my mouth, I mentally glanced ahead at the sentence I wanted to say to see if there was any word I was likely to stutter on.

For me, speaking was like riding down a highway and reading aloud from a series of billboards. I knew that to speak normally I had to keep moving forward at a steady pace. Yet every once in a while I became aware of an obstacle, like an enormous boulder, blocking the road some five or six billboards ahead of me. I knew that when I got to that particular word I would be unable to say it. I never figured out why I stuttered on one word rather than another.

Some sounds—like the "m" sound at the beginning of a word—were particularly troublesome; but, even with these, the context was all-important. A sentence might have two words beginning with "m," such as "I'll have to ask my mother." The moment I framed this sentence in my mind, I knew that I would have no trouble pronouncing "my" but that "mother" would be impossible. My usual strategy at such times was to speed up and try to crash through the obstacle. When I succeeded, the sentence came out like this: "I'll (pause for deep breath) havetoaskmymother."

This trick worked just often enough to convince some people that I stuttered because I talked too fast. But when it failed I found myself struck dumb in midsentence, unable to go forward or turn back. There were times when I got as far as the first sound in the difficult word and could do nothing but repeat it like a broken record, in the classic stutter that is imitated—usually for laughs—in books and movies. More often, I had a complete block; I would try to form the first sound in the word and something inside me would snap shut, so that if I opened my mouth nothing came out.

At that point, I usually backed up and looked for a detour. Sometimes all I had to do was find a less troublesome word that meant the same thing. For example, I might be able to get away with something like "I'll have to check with my folks." If I couldn't think of a synonym quickly enough, I had no choice but to rephrase the sentence, to try to sneak up on the difficult word from 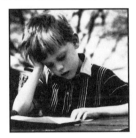 another direction; the result might come out as… "You know how mothers are, I better ask her first."

I didn't have the slightest idea why the same word should be easier to say in one context than in another, but whenever it worked out that way I felt absurd pride in my accomplishment; no one else knew that in order to speak with any fluency I had to become a kind of walking thesaurus. But the strategies of substitution and circumlocution created their own problems. The farther I strayed from the original wording of the sentence, the more I had to guard against letting subtle changes of meaning creep in.

If I wasn't careful, I could find myself saying things I didn't quite mean, just to be able to say something. In a way, my situation was not so different from that of a writer in a totalitarian country who tries to communicate under the constant threat of censorship. The fact that I carried the censor around inside my head did not make the situation any less oppressive.

(This last quotation comes from the book "Stuttering, The Disorder of Many Theories" by Gerald Jones, published by Farrar, Straus & Giroux.)

Some Final Thoughts about Stuttering

Having recently experienced congestive heart failure and informed that I should put my affairs in order, I find an urge to summarize what I have learned about stuttering in 85 years.

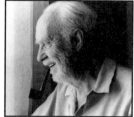

When I was a youth of sixteen I swore an oath to a birch sapling that I would devote my life to finding the cause and cure of stuttering. Decade after decade I returned to that tree and confessed I had found neither. That birch tree died a long time ago but if it were still living I would have to say the same thing today.

I have known thousands of stutterers and have studied the disorder in them and in myself. I have done research and written much about the disorder. I have read most of the world literature. I have explored most of the different kinds of treatment, have helped many to untangle their tongues, and have failed to help others. What then are my final conclusions about stuttering? I believe:

- That stuttering is essentially a neuromuscular disorder whose core consists of tiny lags and disruptions in the timing of the complicated movements required for speech.

- That the usual response to these lags is an automatic part word repetition or prolongation.

- That some children, because of heredity or as yet unknown brain pathology, have more of these than others do.

- That most children who begin to stutter become fluent perhaps because of maturation or because they do not react to their lags, repetitions, or prolongations by struggle or avoidance.

- That those who do struggle or avoid because of frustration or penalties will probably continue to stutter all the rest of their lives no matter what kind of therapy they receive.

- That these struggle and avoidance behaviors are learned and can be modified and unlearned though the lags cannot.

- That the goal of therapy for the confirmed stutterer should not be a reduction in the number of dysfluencies or zero stuttering. Fluency-enhancing procedures can easily result in stutter-free speech temporarily but maintaining it is almost impossible. The stutterer already knows how to be fluent. What he doesn't know is how to stutter. He can be taught to stutter so easily and briefly that he can have very adequate communication skills. Moreover, when he discovers he can stutter without struggle or avoidance most of his frustration and other negative emotion will subside.

Have I anything more to say? Yes, that I still have hope that sooner or later others will fulfill the vow I made to that birch tree. Meanwhile I wish to testify that it is possible to live a happy and useful life even though you stutter.

Charles Van Riper

For more information about stuttering:

Advice to Those Who Stutter

Offers practical advice written by twenty-eight men and women speech pathologists who themselves stutter, advising what helped them and what they believe will help anyone who stutters control his or her difficulty.

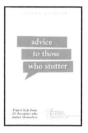

Publication No. 0009   116 pages

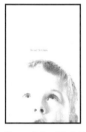

If Your Child Stutters: A Guide for Parents

An authoritative and understandable book for parents. Contains examples of what to do to help the disfluent child. Can be used as a supplement to clinical advice.

Publication No. 0011   64 pages

Translated versions also available:

Spanish: Publication No. 0015   French: Publication No. 0017

Do You Stutter: A Guide for Teens

Because you are a teen and because you sometimes stutter, some problems are uniquely yours. This book is written to and for you in the hope of helping you solve some of these problems. Each chapter is written by a specialist in the field of stuttering.

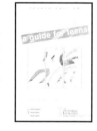

Publication No. 0021   80 pages

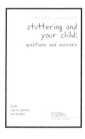

Stuttering and Your Child: Questions and Answers

For parents, teachers and all those wanting to help the child who stutters. Is often used as a supplement to clinical treatment. Written by seven leading authorities.

Publication No. 0022   64 pages

Sometimes I Just Stutter

A book for children between the ages of 7 and 12. This new book has information on teasing, letters to family members and teachers, why stuttering varies day to day, and a wealth of other information.

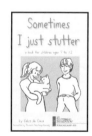

Publication No. 0031   40 pages
Spanish Version No. 0032

Glossary

Many speech pathology words are listed in this glossary which are not used in the book. These are inserted for the education of readers who may not be familiar with the meanings of expressions frequently used in books about stuttering.

accent. The components of increased stress, loudness, or emphasis placed on certain syllables in a word, or group of words. Accent may also be related to *linguistic stress* and "dialect." (See *prosody.*)

acceptance approach. Based on the hypothesis that although stutterers may not have a choice as to whether or not they stutter, they do have a choice as to how they stutter. Accordingly, stuttering can be fully accepted, since it is possible to stutter in a variety of ways, including *fluent stuttering.*

accessory behaviors (secondary behaviors or symptoms). The abnormal actions and behaviors exhibited by the stutterer in attempting to avoid and/or escape from the *core behaviors* of stuttering. *Avoidance behaviors* include such things as pausing, *postponing,* using gestural *timing devices* or verbal *starters,* and trying to *disguise* the stuttering. *Escape behaviors* used to *interrupt* the stuttering and gain release from moments of stuttering include movements such as eye blinks, arm swinging, grimaces, head and jaw jerks, finger snapping, throat clearing and hand/finger tapping, etc.

acquired stuttering. Neurogenic-Acquired Stuttering: As differentiated from "developmental stuttering," this refers to the stuttering-like behaviors in children, adolescents or adults following damage to the central nervous system (CNS) in persons who have no prior history of stuttering. The onset of neurogenic (acquired) stuttering is usually sudden. Causes include head trauma, stroke, anoxia, tumor and drug use. Often co-occurs with features found in aphasia, and dysarthria.

Psychogenic-Acquired stuttering: As differentiated from "developmental stuttering," this has been used to refers to stuttering acquired during adulthood which is at least partially a post-stress response to chronic or acute psychological disturbances in persons who have no prior history of stuttering. It has also been used to refer to document cases of stuttering associated with a conversion reaction. The onset of psychogenic (acquired) stuttering is usually sudden, and related to significant events associated with extreme psychological stress.

adaptation effect. A temporary reduction in the frequency and/or severity of stuttering behaviors resulting from repeated oral readings of the same or highly similar verbal material. Adaptation is sometimes measured in terms of the observed frequency of stuttering during successive readings of the same passage.

In addition to a reduction in the frequency of stuttering there is often a concomitant reduction in associated effort (tension-struggle) and duration of moments of stuttering.

adjacency effect. During repeated oral readings of the same material, when the previously stuttered words have been omitted from the passage, there is a tendency for stuttering to occur on words that are adjacent to where stuttering previously occurred during the earlier readings.

advertising. Clinical programs that emphasize helping the stutterer learn to cope with stuttering and become desensitized to stuttering ask the client to advertise his stuttering by doing a lot of *voluntary stuttering* in public.

affective reactions. Affective reactions are the feelings and emotions that the stutterer experiences during the time period before, during, and after the moment of stuttering. Affective reactions also appear to be related to feelings of denial and/or *avoidance*. Prior to stuttering the person may experience anticipation and apprehension ranging from minimal awareness up to devastating fear and panic; during the moment of stuttering there may be a sense of detachment and confusion or "mental blankness" and a lack of "contact with the self." Following release from the moment of stuttering there may be feelings of *shame, guilt,* embarrassment and feelings of anxiety over the fact that stuttering may occur again.

airflow management. A clinical approach wherein the stutterer attempts to integrate a long, relaxed, passive sigh with the slow initiation of the first syllable of a word in order to maintain air flow by reducing tension and pressure within the vocal track.

anticipatory behaviors. Those behaviors in which the stutterer engages in an attempt to *avoid, disguise* or otherwise prevent stuttering.

anticipatory emotions. Those anticipatory feelings, emotions or attitudinal reactions that result from the stutterer's dread of feared sounds, words, situations or interpersonal relationships.

anticipatory struggle. The anticipatory-struggle hypothesis, which permits a wide array of etiological possibilities, suggests that stuttering involves both the prior anticipation and expectation that speech is a difficult task to perform, as well as the tensions, *fragmentations* and struggle (effort) associated with attempts to gain release from the moment of stuttering itself.

aphasia. The partial or complete loss of the receptive and/or expressive use of language as a result of damage to the central nervous system. Persons suffering from expressive aphasia (e.g., nonfluent aphasia) frequently have problems maintaining speech fluency, but this is considered a fluency disorder which is different from stuttering. These patients frequently experience word finding and word retrieval problems and often compensate for this difficulty with word *substitutions* and *circumlocutions*.

approach-avoidance conflict. This term describes the conflict which the stutterer experiences as he approaches a feared word or situation. His desire for *avoidance* of verbal difficulty struggles for mastery against his desire for speaking, and the conflict may be expressed *overtly* in stuttering behaviors that interfere with speaking. The stutterer is caught in a conflict where he wants to talk and communicate but wants to avoid stuttering: at the same time, he wants to not stutter, but not abandon communication.

approximation. As used in operant conditioning and learning, the reward or positive reinforcement given to productions that come progressively or successively closer and closer to the desired target. In stuttering, this is used to refer to deliberate attempts on the part of the stutterer to speak in a manner that comes successively closer and closer to the desired target.

articulation. Literally, a joining: in speech, the utterance of the individual sounds of speech in connected discourse; the movements during speech of the organs that modify the stream of voiced and unvoiced breath in meaningful sounds: The speech function performed largely through movements of the mandible, lips, tongue and soft palate.

auditory feedback. As related to the self-monitoring of one's own speech through self-hearing. (See *feedback, delayed auditory feedback.)*

avoidance behaviors. Actions or patterns of behavior which the stutterer uses in trying to avoid difficulty. These include abnormal variations employed such as *postponements,* word *substitutions, circumlocutions,* vocalized or nonvocalized pauses, or the complete refusal to speak. Such maneuvers usually tend to increase any fear of difficulty the stutterer may have. Unlike the *escape behaviors* that occur during the moment of stuttering itself in an attempt to permit release, *avoidance* behaviors occur prior to the moment of stuttering in an attempt to totally prevent its occurrence.

behavior modification. A general term for any of a variety of clinical procedures based on *learning theory* and *conditioning* principles. Such procedures are used both to modify the disruptive negative emotional responses of the stutterer to words and situations, and to reduce the maladaptive *avoidance* and *escape behaviors* that confirmed stutterers tend to display.

between-word disfluencies. Listeners make perceptual judgments of disfluency and stuttering, and sometimes it is helpful to determine whether disfluencies occur *within words* or between words. *Within word disfluencies* such as sound or syllable *repetitions, prolongations, disrhythmic phonations* and *tense pauses* are more apt to be considered "stuttered" and represent a greater danger sign than disfluencies that occur in between words such as *interjections, revisions,* phrase repetitions and multisyllabic whole-word repetitions.

biofeedback. The measurement of physical activity and the display of this activity to the user in real-time so that the person can develop awareness and control of the activity. Some clinical programs make use of biofeedback to help the stutterer modify the activities needed for fluent speech production: e.g., respiration, phonation and articulation.

blending. A technique in which the stutterer gradually shifts from one part of the sound or syllable into the next.

block. One of several types of stuttering in which the *fixation (closure)* is total. The flow of speech is obstructed completely at any one, or several locations: larynx, lips, tongue, etc. The abnormality is perceived by the listener through visual awareness that the person is attempting to speak, even though little or no sound is heard. Some people use this term to refer to any type of stuttering moment. (See *tonic block: clonic block.*)

bounce. A stuttering pattern in which there are voluntary repetitions, usually of the first syllable of the word, as in "base-base-base-ball."

cancellation. The technique used in therapy of responding to the occurrence of a moment of stuttering by a deliberate pause followed by a second attempt on the word in which a different and more fluent form of stuttering is used. This consists of coming to a complete halt after the stuttered word has been finally uttered, pausing a moment and then attempting to say the word again with less struggle and *avoidance*. This does not imply that on the second trial the stutterer is to be fluent; rather, he should attempt a modified and easier form of stuttering. This procedure is called *post-block correction* by some clinicians.

carryover. Procedures designed to assist the stutterer in *transferring* and *maintaining* newly learned speech therapy techniques to everyday situations.

classical conditioning. A form of conditioning in which a previously neutral stimulus is paired with an *unconditioned stimulus*. In time, the neutral stimulus becomes conditioned, and elicits a *conditioned response* which is similar to the unconditioned response originally elicited by the unconditioned stimulus. (Synonyms: Pavlovian conditioning, respondent conditioning, reflex conditioning.) (See *conditioned stimulus.*)

clinician, (speech-language). See *speech-language pathologist.*

cluttering. A disorder of both speech and language processing that frequently results in rapid, *disrhythmic*, sporadic, unorganized, and often unintelligible speech. Additional problems include *repetition* of sounds, syllables, words and phrases, false starts and revisions, sequencing errors, word retrieval problems, run-on sentences and the excessively fast and irregular production of syllables. Persons who clutter usually have great difficulty with self-monitoring.

conditioned response. After the repeated paring of a *neutral stimulus* with an unconditioned stimulus, the *neutral stimulus* becomes a *conditioned stimulus,* and elicits a conditioned response.

conditioned stimulus. A previously *neutral stimulus,* after contiguous pairing with an unconditioned stimulus, takes on properties similar to the original unconditioned stimulus and has the ability to elicit a *conditioned response* that is similar to the original unconditioned response.

conditioning. The process of acquiring, establishing, learning, modifying, or extinguishing behavioral and/or emotional responses. Forms of conditioning include: *classical* (Pavlovian, respondent, reflex) conditioning; *counter conditioning; operant* (Skinnerian, instrumental) conditioning; *vicarious conditioning; deconditioning.* When a response that formerly occurred only rarely or not at all is "conditioned" to occur more frequently, learning is assumed to have taken place, provided that the change is relatively long lasting. Conditioning may occur by chance, or by conscious manipulation of antecedent stimuli and/or contingent consequences.

consonant. A conventional speech sound other than a vowel, and characterized by constriction or total *closure* at one or more points along the vocal tract. Can be voiced or unvoiced.

constitutional origin. The theory that some stutterers possess, or possessed at the time of onset, a "physical or genetic difference," or malfunctioning of the nervous system, which was sufficient to create, under stress, disruptions in the fluent flow of speech.

continuous phonation. As a means of maintaining fluency, some clinicians suggest that the stutterer maintain voicing throughout the production of the utterance. This produces an effect whereby the duration of the sounds and syllables is increased by degrees that can range from minimal to extreme. A similar effect can result from the use of *Delayed Auditory Feedback.*

core behaviors (core features). Most researchers and clinicians differentiate between the core features of stuttering and the *accessory (secondary)* features that develop as a means of avoiding and/or escaping from the core features. Core features are generally thought to include the *repetition* of sounds, syllables and single-syllable words; the vocalized and nonvocalized sound *prolongation,* and complete stoppages due to *tense pauses, hard contacts* and *silent blocks.* In the early developmental stages of stuttering these "core features" are easy, effortless and relaxed: later, however, they coexist with *accessory behaviors* when they are accompanied by effort, tension, and struggle.

covert features. Unlike the overt behaviors of stuttering which can be seen and/or heard and are relatively easy to measure in terms of their frequency, intensity, duration, and type, the covert behaviors are not openly shown and less easily determined. They include such cognitive and emotional factors as fear, anxiety, negative emotion, *shame, guilt* and frustration, etc. These "concealed or invisible" features are often difficult to determine. (See *interiorized stuttering.*)

delayed auditory feedback (DAF). When speaking under conditions of delayed auditory feedback, we hear what we have said a short time after we have said it. Most normally fluent speakers become highly disfluent when exposed to DAF and many stutterers experience decreased stuttering under DAF. DAF can also be used clinically both to help establish fluency as well as control/modify the stuttering.

Demands and Capacities Model. This model states that stuttering is likely to occur when demands for fluent and continuous speech exceed the child's capacities to perform at a level required by these demands. Factors that affect fluent speech include (1) motoric coordination, (2) linguistic ability, (3) social and emotional functioning, and (4) cognitive development. Clinically, attempts are made to reduce demands placed upon the child and increase the child's capacities for dealing with them.

desensitization. Desensitization generally takes place at two levels: emotional and behavioral. Emotionally, desensitization therapy attempts to help the client feel increasingly relaxed and comfortable in situations that previously were associated with fear, anxiety and other forms of negative emotion. Behaviorally, desensitization attempts to help the client tolerate periods of physical tension during moments of stuttering accompanied by tension and struggle. To accomplish desensitization, stutterers are often exposed to a hierarchy of increasingly stressful situations where they work to remain calm and relaxed in activities such as *voluntary stuttering, pseudo-stuttering* or faking.

developmental disfluencies/developmental hesitations. The developmental repetitions, prolongations and stumblings in the speech of children learning to talk. In the natural development of speech, while learning to talk, most children's speech is marked by effortless developmental hesitations to some extent. Included in this category are word and phrase repetitions and such *accessory* vocalizations as the *Interjection* of "um" and "ah." These "normal developmental" hesitations are particularly common during times of linguistic stress, which is a part of language learning, and situational stress under conditions of situational and interpersonal difficulty.

diagnosogenic theory. The theory that "stuttering" as a clinical problem and as a definite disorder, was found to occur not before being diagnosed but after being diagnosed. According to this theory, the problem of stuttering arises when a listener, usually a parent, evaluates or classifies or diagnoses the child's developmental hesitations, *repetitions,* and *prolongations* as stuttering, and reacts to them as a consequence with concern and disapproval. As the child senses this concern and disapproval he reacts by speaking more hesitantly and with concern of his own, and finally, with the tensions and struggle involved in efforts to keep from hesitating or *repeating.*

disflyency (dysfluency). Used interchangeably by some clinicians and differentially by others. Some feel that the prefix "dys-" should be used where there is reasonable suspicion of "organicity" to warrant the more medical terminology. The prefix "dis-" is used to denote mislearning and more psycho-emotional components. Other clinicians opt for the term "nonfluency." In any event, the terms refer to speech which is not smooth or fluent. All speakers talk disfluently at times; i.e., they hesitate or stumble in varying degrees. All stutterers are disfluent, but not all disfluency is stuttering. For instance, "disfluency" could describe the developmental hesitations of a child learning to talk, or the disrhythmic breaks in the speech of an adult. Other disfluencies are associated with neuropathology such as the speech characteristics associated with apraxia, parkinsonism, multiple sclerosis, myesthenia gravis and others.

distraction. The diversion of attention: filling the mind with thoughts of other things so that the expectancy of stuttering is minimized. Keeping the *anticipatory emotions* of stuttering from consciousness, thus temporarily affecting release from fear of stuttering and the act of stuttering.

dysphonia. Impairment of the voice, manifested by hoarseness, breathiness or other defects of *phonation* due to organic, functional or psychogenic causes.

176

easy onset (gentle onset). Starting the voicing of a sound, syllable or word at a slow, smooth rate. The *duration* of each syllable within a word is stretched for up to two seconds. The easy onset is relaxed, and produced without effort: also referred to as gentle onset.

escape behaviors. The behavioral reactions of a stutterer to release, *interrupt* or otherwise escape from a moment of stuttering. Since escape behaviors allow release from the unpleasant, aversive or noxious stimulus of stuttering, they are *negatively reinforced* and tend to persist.

extrovert. A person whose attention and interests are largely directed toward what is outside the self; one primarily interested in social or group activities and practical affairs; contrasted with "introvert."

eye contact. Looking the listener in the eye while talking to him. Generally a natural, although not a constant interaction, of the speaker's eyes with the listener's eyes. Maintaining eye contact is considered a technique in stuttering therapy recommended to help the stutterer combat feelings of *shame,* embarrassment or inadequacy.

fear. The apprehension of unpleasantness which arises when the stutterer consciously perceives situations which lead him to anticipate difficulty talking. This fear of difficulty may be and often is intense. It can and sometimes does temporarily paralyze thought and action. Stuttering is usually relatively proportionate to the amount of fear present. Stuttering fears may be of persons, of sounds or words, or of situations such as talking in groups or on the telephone, etc.

feared word/feared sound. This term refers to a word or sound upon which the stutterer anticipates difficulty. Stutterers frequently attempt to avoid feared words and sounds by word *substitutions, circumlocutions* or paraphrasing the utterance.

feedback. The process of modifying one's own responses based on either internal or external cues. Returning a portion of the output of a transmitted signal as input for self regulation. The reinforcing effect of the stutterer's auditory or proprioceptive perceptions of his own speech. (Also see *corrective feedback* and *delayed auditory feedback.*)

fixation. The maintenance of an articulatory or phonatory posture for an abnormal duration; the temporary arresting of the speech muscles in a rigid position. The airway is abnormally constricted, but not completely blocked. Fixations typically result in the production of sounds which may be both audible and vocalized (vvvvvine) or audible but not vocalized (fffffine.)

fluency. Fluent speech involves the ability to talk with normal levels of *continuity, rate, rhythm* and effort. Fluency involves the smoothness with which units of speech (sounds, syllables, words, phrases) flow together. Fluent speech flows easily and is usually made without effort. Abnormally broken, slow, or effortful speech is not fluent.

fluency shaping. Fluency shaping therapy is usually based on operant conditioning and programming principles; e.g., breath stream management, successive approximations, reinforcement of fluency targets such as fluency enhancing behaviors, etc. Some form of fluency is first established in a controlled stimulus situation. This fluency is reinforced and gradually modified to approximate normal conversational speech in the clinical setting. This speech is then transferred to the person's daily speaking environment.

frustration tolerance. The capacity of the stutterer to resist feelings of frustration because of his inability to speak without difficulty; the ability to put up with or endure the communication handicaps resulting from not being able to talk freely.

genetic. Inherited, as determined through genes, but not necessarily congenitally present at birth. Some persons believe that stuttering, or at least some stuttering subtypes, may have an etiologic (causative) basis in genetically inherited traits, tendencies or predispositions.

group therapy. The counseling of and among stutterers in a group, including the use of speech within such a social situation. The interchange of feelings, ideas and discussions about stuttering problems in a group gives the stutterer emotional release and helps him to develop better insights and understanding through a knowledge of how others react to their problems.

hard contact. The result of tightness or tension in the muscles of the tongue and/or lips and/or jaw, etc., when the stutterer fears and attempts to say plosive consonant sounds such as p, b, t, d, k, g.

in-block correction. This refers to a process the stutterer goes through to correct the production of a stuttered word while he is stuttering on it. See *pull-out.*

incidence. The incidence of stuttering refers to how many people have stuttered at some time in their lives. Although researchers have used different methodologies to gather these data, and since they have used slightly different definitions of stuttering, it is estimated that about 5% of the population have experienced periods of stuttering lasting longer than six months. Estimates of incidence, inclusive of children who may have evidenced periods of stuttering lasting for only a short time period, are as high as 15%. (See *prevalence.*)

inhibition. Restraint on one's ability to act by either conscious or subconscious processes: the partial checking or complete blocking of one impulse or mental process by another nearly simultaneous impulse or mental process. The fear of stuttering tends to inhibit the stutterer's impulse or desire to speak.

introvert. An inward oriented personality; one who prefers his own thoughts and activities to association with others; one primarily interested or preoccupied with self. Contrasted with *extrovert.*

labial. Pertaining to the lips; speech sounds requiring the use of the lip or lips such as "p, m, f, v."

larynx. The primary source of *phonation* resulting from vocal fold vibration; the "voice box" which houses the vocal folds. Located at the top of the trachea, below the bone or bones which support the tongue and its muscles.

laterality theory. Refers to the theory that a shift in handedness or confused cerebral dominance is a factor in the cause or in the maintenance of stuttering. According to this theory, the use of the non-preferred hand in written and other skilled activities contributes to a cerebral instability affecting speech control in such a way as to generate stuttering. Laterality theory refers to insufficiently established dominance of one cerebral hemisphere over another.

learned behavior. Any relatively permanent change in a person's behavior resulting from his reaction to or interaction with environmental influences or from reinforced practice: an acquired neuro-muscular, verbal, emotional, or other type of response to certain stimuli.

light contact. Loose, relaxed or non-tense contacts of the lips and/or tongue on plosive sounds. Contacts of the lips and/or tongue which are optimal for the production of speech sounds as contrasted to the hard, tense contacts which are often a part of a stuttering pattern.

maintenance. In stuttering usually refers to the continuation of improvement as related to the effectiveness of treatment. Procedures for keeping a desired learned behavior at a high level of frequency, e.g., procedures for preventing relapse.

masking. An interference with perception of a sound or pattern of sounds by simultaneously presenting another of a different frequency, intensity, quality, or pattern to one or both ears of the subject. Masking is usually presented via head phones and is used to interfere with the stutterer's perception of his own voice. The usual effect, especially at sufficiently high levels of loudness, is increased fluency.

modifying the stuttering pattern. Refers to the stutterer changing what he does when he stutters. Clinicians suggest that the stutterer can deliberately change his stuttering behavior and learn to stutter in an easier manner. Clinical emphasis is reducing the overall severity of the stuttering rather than replacing it with fluent speech. In so modifying his stuttering pattern he learns to change his way of speaking and develop a style of talking which is less abnormal and free of excessive tensing. A basic fact revealed by laboratory and clinical studies is that the behavior called stuttering is modifiable. (See *slide, pull-out, proprioceptive monitoring, easy onset, cancellation, preparatory set.*)

monitoring. A self-observation technique in which the stutterer seeks to become highly aware of the articulatory movements of his speech, as well as other behaviors which make up his characteristic and habitual pattern of stuttering. This would include continuous self-observation of the crutches and tricks he uses in his act of stuttering.

monotone. Voice characterized by little or no variation of pitch or loudness.

179

neurosis. A personality disorder generally characterized by anxiety, phobias, obsessions or compulsions which are irrational but nevertheless real to the possessor, and which are probably caused by interpersonal conflict. There is no gross personality disorganization, and there may not be any behavioral manifestations. Neurosis is a mental disorder that prevents the victim from dealing effectively with reality.

objective attitude. Referring to the attitude that it is desirable for the stutterer to have toward his stuttering; a feeling relatively independent of one's personal prejudices or apprehensions and not distorted by *shame* or embarrassment; the *acceptance* of his stuttering as a problem rather than a curse.

onset. The onset of stuttering usually occurs during childhood, with some cases of developmental stuttering occurring up through the time of puberty. The median age at onset is at about age four. Onset occurring after puberty is usually attributable to extreme cases of physical or psychological trauma.

operant conditioning. The process by which the frequency of a response may be changed as a result of controlling its consequences. There are a variety of procedures in which a clinician can arrange for contingent stimulation to occur following a response. If the consequence is positive, the response (acquisition) should increase in frequency; if the consequence is negative, the response should decrease (extinction). This process is often theorized to be the way in which the voluntary behaviors of *avoidance* and *escape* are learned. Behaviorists consider this as the basic strategy for achieving behavior change. (Synonym: *instrumental conditioning,* Skinnerian conditioning.) (See *conditioning.*)

oscillation(s). In stuttering, the *tremorous* vibrations or repetitions of speech muscle movements temporarily interfering with ongoing speech, as opposed to the fixation or prolongation of an articulatory sound or posture.

overt behavior. Clearly visible and/or audible behavior. The opposite of *covert.*

pantomime. The art of conveying a thought or story by expressive bodily movements. As part of *cancellation,* some clinicians ask the stutterer to pantomime the moment of stuttering in order to identify its components and aid in *desensitization.*

phobia. An excessive and objectively inappropriate degree of fear or dread. An anxiety reaction that is focused on a particular object or situation.

phonation. Vocalization; the act or process of producing voice; production of the voiced sounds of speech by means of vocal fold vibration.

pitch. The listener's perception of the highness or lowness of sounds depending on the frequency of the vocal fold vibrations.

play therapy. The use of play activities in psychotherapy or speech therapy with children, in which the child is given opportunities, within defined limits, for the free expression of socially or personally unacceptable feelings in the presence of an accepting therapist. In individual play therapy sessions the therapist may observe the child as he plays with materials (such as puppets, clay or toys) permitting him within reason to freely express emotional feelings and conflicts for purposes of catharsis or insight.

plosive. A speech sound made by impounding the air stream momentarily until pressure has been developed and then suddenly released, as in "p,b,t,d,k,g."

post-block correction. This is a process the stutterer goes through to correct the production of a stuttered word after he has stuttered on it. See *cancellation.*

postponement behaviors. Any behavior or technique used to avoid stuttering by pausing, delaying or stalling the attempt to produce a feared sound or word in the hope that the fear will subside enough to allow production.

pre-block correction. This is a process the stutterer goes through to prepare to produce a word on which he expects to stutter. See *preparatory set.*

preparatory set. The anticipatory response to the conditioned stimuli of an anticipated act of stuttering. The *covert* rehearsal behavior of the stutterer which he uses in getting ready for the difficulty which he anticipates. This procedure is called the *pre-block correction* by some clinicians.

primary stuttering. The label sometimes used to describe the speech of a young child when it is marked by repetitions and/or hesitations or prolongations which the observer regards as abnormal, but which do not seem to embarrass the child nor does the child seem to feel that these disfluencies constitute a difficulty or abnormality. Such disfluent speech occurs during the growth and development of the child's ability to talk and may be observed to increase when the child is under certain kinds of emotional or communicative or linguistic stress. Many clinicians protest labeling such speech as stuttering, although it may be the beginning stage of a stuttering problem.

prolongation. As related to stuttering, the involuntary lengthening or prolonging of vocalized speech sounds (rrrrunning, aaaapple), or nonvocalized sounds (sssseven, ffffourteen). Sometimes refers to prolongation of an articulatory position, as when the person stops completely and holds his mouth in the position to say "p<pause>icture." Prolongations are frequently accompanied by increases in loudness and/or pitch.

As related to therapy, the easy voluntary prolongation of sounds and syllables on feared and nonfeared words is used quite extensively to modify the stuttering pattern. (See *modifying the stuttering pattern; disrhythmic phonation.*)

pseudo-stuttering. Deliberately faked or false stuttering produced to imitate difficultly which a stutterer might experience. Sometimes used to aid in *desensitization.* (See *voluntary stuttering.*)

psychotherapy. The treatment of behavioral or emotional problems, such as stuttering, by counseling, or by reeducating and influencing the person's mental approaches and his ways of thinking, or of evaluating his problems; any procedures intended to improve the condition of a person that are directed at a change in his mental approach to his problems; particularly his attitudes toward himself and his environment.

pull-out. Based on the hypothesis that it is possible for a stutterer to pull out of difficulty during a moment of stuttering, this term refers to a voluntarily controlled, gradual, release from the stuttering moment. In pulling out of blocks, the stutterer does not let the original blocking run its course. Instead he makes a deliberate attempt to modify it before the release occurs and before the word is spoken. This procedure is called *in-block correction* by some clinicians.

rate control. A technique with which the stutterer attempts to speak slowly and deliberately, often with each syllable given equal or nearly equal stress. The extent to which rate control is used to "facilitate fluency" or "repress stuttering" is highly controversial.

regression. As related to *relapse,* having more speech difficulty usually as a result of reverting back to an earlier faulty method of talking.

relapse. Pertaining to *regression.* See this term.

repetition. The repeating of a sound, syllable, word or phrase. Some clinicians differentiate between repetitions which are vocalized (l-l-lit) and nonvocalized (f-f-fit), and whether the syllable is correctly co-articulated (base-base-baseball) or contains the schwa vowel (buh-buh- baseball). Word repetitions may be of single syllable whole words (he-he-he has it) or words of more than one syllable ("David-David-David has it.")

residual air. Generally referred to as the amount of air remaining in the lungs following exhalation.

rhythm. The overall melody, cadence and flow of speech, as influenced by such factors as syllable, stress and rate of articulation.

rhythm method. Attempts to help the stutterer speak fluently by altering the rhythm of speech through such means as singing or speaking in singsong manner, speaking in time with a regularly recurring rhythm such as to the best of a metronome, or timing the speech and syllable gestures to an arm swing.

secondary stuttering. As opposed to primary and transitional stuttering, secondary stuttering is a hesitating or stumbling in uttering words with an awareness that this way of talking is abnormal and constitutes a difficulty; speech interruptions plus *struggle* and *accessory behaviors,* plus *fear* and *avoidance* reactions.

secondary symptoms. The abnormal actions, behaviors and positions exhibited by a stutterer in trying to *escape* speech difficulty. These include movements such as eye blinks, arm swinging, grimaces, head and body jerks, finger snapping, clearing the throat, and hand tapping, etc. These refer to the movements which a stutterer characteristically and abnormally uses when approaching and escaping from a feared word and when *struggling* to release himself from the moment of stuttering. (See *accessory behaviors.*)

semantics. The scientific study of word meanings.

sensitivity. In the case of stutterers, usually refers to the tendency toward being easily upset, embarrassed or otherwise easily affected. Feelings of hypersensitivity may relate to both speech and non speech parameters.

situational fears. Concerns regarding certain places or events in which the speaker expects to have increased stuttering difficulty.

slide. Uttering the different sounds of a syllable with prolonged, slow motion transitions: moving slowly through the syllable or word. In the slide technique the stutterer *prolongs* slightly the initial sound and the transition to the rest of the word, keeping the release as smooth and gradual as possible, and maintaining sound throughout.

spasmodic (spastic) dysphonia. Persons with spasmodic dysphonia experience intermittent blockages of *phonation* resulting from spasms of the adductor or abductor muscles of the larynx resulting in intermittently choked or strangled production of voice. This has been referred to as "stuttering/stammering of the vocal cords," or "laryngeal stuttering."

speech-language pathologist. A person professionally educated in the assessment, prevention and treatment of disorders of articulation, voice, language and fluency. Although terms such as speech correctionist, speech therapist and speech clinician are frequently used, the American Speech-Language-Hearing Association prefers use of the term Speech-Language Pathologist. Academic requirements include a master's degree and the completion of the supervised clinical fellowship year following formal academic course work, and passing a national examination.

speech-language pathology. The science or study of normal and disordered articulation, language, voice and fluency and their diagnosis and treatment.

stammering. Synonymous with "stuttering." (British usage.)

starter. Unlike *stallers* and *postponements, starters* are used to initiate or reinitiate forward movement into an utterance. This may involve the use of a stereotypic phrase such as "well, let me see" or "you know" in order to get a "running start."

stress. Psychologically, an emotional and cognitive factor that causes bodily or mental tension. Physically, as associated with effort, tension or struggle.

struggle behavior. This includes a wide range of *secondary* or *accessory behaviors* performed by the stutterer in attempt to escape from a moment of stuttering. Devices used to *interrupt* and release, involving excessive effort, tension, changes in pitch or loudness, and *escape behaviors* such as head-jerks, eye-blinks, arm movements and jaw jerks, etc.

stuttering. Stuttering is a communication disorder characterized by excessive involuntary disruptions in the smooth and rhythmic flow of speech, particularly when such disruptions consist of *repetitions* or *prolongations* of a sound or syllable, and when they are accompanied by emotions such as fear and anxiety, and behaviors such as *avoidance* and *struggle.*

stuttering pattern. In the case of the individual stutterer, refers to the particular way he experiences difficulty in talking, or the specific things he does and the order in which he does these things that interfere with his speaking; the particular sequence of reactions in his stuttering speech behavior.

syllable. A unit of spoken language consisting of a vowel, usually with one or more consonant sounds preceding and/or following it; v, vc, cv, cvc, ccvc, etc. (i.e., v= vowel c=consonant.)

tension. Mental, emotional, nervous or physical strain, often resulting in unnecessary intensity that disturbs normal functioning of the organs of speech.

therapy. The prevention, early intervention and treatment of any clinically significant condition such as stuttering.

tic. A sudden spasmodic and purposeless movement of some muscle or muscle group, particularly of the face, usually occurring under emotional stress. Possibly organic or psychogenic in origin.

time pressure. At the moment the stutterer is expected to speak he often has an almost panicky feeling of haste and urgency. He feels he is under "time pressure" and with no time to lose, and so he has a somewhat compulsive feeling that he must speak instantly without allowing time for deliberate and relaxed expression.

transfer. The process of generalizing a newly acquired behavior to new and different environments: for example, the transfer of improved fluency from the therapy room to the classroom or to the home or office. Sometimes referred to as "carry-over."

tremor. A localized quivering or vibratory motion of a muscle or muscle group when an articulatory position is suddenly invested with localized hypertension.

vocal cords. Synonymous with vocal folds. The opening and closing of the vocal folds is responsible for the production of laryngeal voicing.

voice. Sound produced by vibration of the vocal folds and modified by the resonators.

voice onset time (VOT). The length of time, measured in milliseconds, between the onset of an external signal such as a tone or light and the initiation of *phonation.*

voluntary stuttering. This may refer to attempts made by the stutterer to imitate or duplicate as closely as possible, or with specific predetermined modifications, his usual, habitual, pattern of stuttering. It may also take the form of easy *prolongations* or relatively spontaneous and effortless *repetitions* of sounds, syllables or the word itself. This style of talking may be used as a deliberate replacement for the usual stuttering behavior and is intended to reduce fear of difficulty by voluntarily doing that which is dreaded. This conscious, purposeful stuttering is also designed to eliminate other avoidance reactions. For the purpose of *desensitization* some clinicians ask the stutterer to add tension and struggle to these voluntary stutterings in order to learn how to better cope with them. (See *pseudo-stuttering*.)

vowel. A voiced speech sound in which the oral part of the breath channel is not blocked and is not constricted enough to cause audible friction: broadly, the most prominent sound in a syllable.

whisper. Speech without vibration of the vocal cords.

Authors of Quotations

★ SOL ADLER, Ph.D.
Professor of Speech Pathology
University of Tennessee,
Knoxville

★ JOSEPH G. AGNELLO, Ph.D.
Professor of Speech Pathology
University of Cincinnati

MERLE ANSBERRY, Ph.D.
*Professor of Emeritus of Speech
Pathology*
University of Hawaii, Honolulu

★ JAMES T. ATEN, Ph.D.
*Chairman of Speech Pathology
Section*
V.A. Hospital, Long Beach,
California

★ DOMINICK A. BARBARA, Ph.D.,
M.D.
Psychiatrist
Karen Horney Clinic, New York
City

★ OLIVER BLOODSTEIN, Ph.D.
Professor of Speech Pathology
Brooklyn College, City University
of New York

★ C. S. BLUEMEL, M.D.
*Late Fellow of the American
Psychiatric Association
and the American College of
Physicians*

★ RICHARD M. BOEHMLER, Ph.D.
Professor of Speech Pathology
University of Montana, Missoula

★ JOHN L. BOLAND, Ph.D.
Clinical Psychiatrist
Oklahoma Psychological and
Educational Center,
Oklahoma City

★ DORVAN BREITENFELDT, Ph.D.
Professor of Speech Pathology
Eastern Washington University

★ SPENCER F. BROWN, Ph.D., M.D.
*formerly Associate Professor of
Pediatrics*
University of Iowa, Iowa City

EDWARD G. CONTURE, Ph.D.
Professor of Speech Pathology
Vanderbilt University, Nashville

★ PAUL R. CZUCHNA, M.A.
Director of Stuttering Programs
Western Michigan University,
Kalamazoo

DENNIS DRAYNA, Ph.D.
*Senior Fellow, National Institute
on Deafness &
Other Communicative
Disorders*
National Institutes of Health

★ LON L. EMERICK, Ph.D.
Professor of Speech Pathology
Northern Michigan University,
Marquette

★ HENRY FREUND, M.D.
*Fellow, American Psychiatric
Association*
Milwaukee, Wisconsin

★ SCOTT GARLAND, M.D.
Occupational Medicine
Winston-Salem, North Carolina

★ HUGO H. GREGORY, M.D.
*Professor and Head, Speech and
Language Pathology*
Northwestern University,
Evanston, Illinois

★ BARRY E. GUITAR, Ph.D.
*Associate Professor, Speech
Pathology*
University of Vermont,
Burlington

★ LLOYD M. HULIT, Ph.D.
Associate *Professor of Speech
Pathology*
Illinois State University, Normal

★ GERALD F. JOHNSON, Ph.D.
Professor of Speech Pathology
University of Wisconsin, Stevens
Point

★ Authorities who have been stutterers.

★ WENDELL JOHNSON, Ph.D.
*formerly Professor of Speech
Pathology and
Director of Speech Clinic*
University of Iowa, Iowa City

★ ALAN G. KAMHI, Ph.D.
*Assistant Professor of Speech
Pathology*
University of Memphis, Memphis,
Tennessee

★ GARY N. LaPORTE, M.A.
*formerly Coordinator of Speech
Pathology Programs*
University of Tampa, Florida

★ HAROLD L. LUPER, Ph.D.
*formerly Professor and Head,
Speech Pathology Department*
University of Tennessee,
Knoxville

★ GERALD A. MAGUIRE, M.D.
*Associate Professor of Clinical
Psychiatry*
University of California, Irvine
School of Medicine

★ FREDERICK MARTIN, M.D.
*formerly Superintendent of
Speech Corrections*
New York City Schools

★ GERALD R. MOSES, Ph.D.
*Associate Professor of Speech
Pathology*
Eastern Michigan University,
Ypsilanti

★ FREDERICK P. MURRAY, Ph.D.
*formerly Director, Division of
Speech Pathology*
University of New Hampshire,
Durham

★ MARGARET M. NEELY, Ph.D.
*Director, Baton Rouge Speech and
Hearing Foundation*
Baton Rouge, Louisiana

WILLIAM H. PERKINS, Ph.D.
*Director, Intensive Therapy
Program for Stuttering*
University of Southern
California, Los Angeles

★ Authorities who have been stutterers.

★ THEODORE J. PETERS, Ph.D.
Professor of Speech Pathology
University of Wisconsin, Eau
Claire

★ MARGARET RAINEY, Ph.D.
Director, Speech Pathology
Shorewood Public Schools,
Wisconsin

★ PETER R. RAMIG, Ph.D.
Professor of Speech Pathology
University of Colorado, Boulder

PETER ROSENBERGER, M.D.
Director, Learning Disorders Unit
Massachusetts General Hospital,
Harvard Medical School, Boston

★ JOSEPH G. SHEEHAN, Ph.D.
Professor of Psychology
University of California, Los
Angeles

★ HAROLD B. STARBUCK, Ph.D.
*Distinguished Service Emeritus
Professor of Speech Pathology*
State University College,
Geneseo, New York

★ COURTNEY STROMSTA, Ph.D.
Professor of Speech Pathology
Western Michigan University,
Kalamazoo

★ WILLIAM D. TROTTER, Ph.D.
*Director, Communicative
Disorders*
Marquette University, Milwaukee

★ CHARLES VAN RIPER, Ph.D.
*Distinguished Professor Emeritus
of Speech Pathology*
Western Michigan University,
Kalamazoo

★ RONALD T. VINNARD, M.D.
The Center for Fluent Speech
Madera, California

★ CONRAD WEDBERG, M.A.
*formerly Director of Speech
Therapy*
Alhambra City Schools,
California

★ DEAN WILLIAMS, Ph.D.
Professor of Speech Pathology
University of Iowa, Iowa City

★ J. DAVID WILLIAMS, Ph.D.
Professor of Speech Pathology
Northern Illinois University,
DeKalb

187

Most of the quotations used in this book came from the following publications:

A Clinician's Guide to Stuttering; Sol Adler
(Charles C. Thomas).

Questions and Answers on Stuttering; Dominick A. Barbara (Charles C. Thomas).

The Riddle of Stuttering; C. S. Bluemel
(Interstate Publishing).

Speech Motor Control in Normal and Disordered Speech; B. Maassen, R. D. Kent, H.F.M. Peters, P.H.H.M. van Lieshout & W. Hulstjin, Eds. (Oxford University Press).

Stuttering, A Second Symposium; Jon Eisenson, Ed.
(Harper & Row).

An Analysis of Stuttering; Emerick and Hamre, Ed.
(Interstate Publishing).

Psychopathology and the Problems of Stuttering;
Henry Freund (Charles C. Thomas).

Controversies About Stuttering Therapy; Hugo Gregory, Ed. (University Park Press).

Learning Theory and Stuttering Therapy; Hugo Gregory, Ed.
(Northwestern University Press).

People in Quandaries; Wendell Johnson (Harper & Brothers).

Stuttering and What You Can Do About It; Wendell Johnson (University of Minnesota Press).

A Stutterer's Story; Frederick Pemberton Murray
(Stuttering Foundation of America).

Stuttering, Research and Therapy; Joseph Sheehan, Ed.
(Harper & Brothers).

Handbook of Speech Pathology; Lee Edward Travis, Ed. (Appleton-Century-Crofts).

Speech Correction; Charles Van Riper (Prentice-Hall).

The Nature of Stuttering; Charles Van Riper (Prentice-Hall).

The Treatment of Stuttering; Charles Van Riper (Prentice-Hall).

Speech Therapy, A Book of Readings; Charles Van Riper, Ed. (Prentice-Hall).

The Stutterer Speaks; Conrad Wedberg (Expression Co.),

and from the publications of the Stuttering Foundation of America.

Index

If you believe this book has helped you or you wish to help this worthwhile cause, please send a donation to:

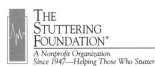

THE
STUTTERING
FOUNDATION®
A Nonprofit Organization
Since 1947—Helping Those Who Stutter

P.O. Box 11749 • Memphis, TN 38111-0749

800-992-9392   901-761-0343

www.stutteringhelp.org

The Stuttering Foundation of America is a tax-exempt organization under section 501(c)(3) of the Internal Revenue Code and is classified as a private operating foundation as defined in section 4942(j)(3). Charitable contributions and bequests to the Foundation are tax-deductible, subject to limitations under the Code.